Young Adult Type 1 Diabetes Realities

Nicole Johnson, DrPH, MPH, MA

Miss America 1999 and T1D since 1993

CONTENTS

INTRODUCTION

Nothing about being a young adult with diabetes is easy. Living with type 1 diabetes (T1D) can prompt insecurity, isolation, and pessimism. It especially torments teens and young adults. The transition from dependence to independence offers an opportunity to define one's persona and self-image. It is a chance to decide who you are and how others will see you. This includes the question of disclosure of T1D. The newness of independence can also highlight challenges for those who have always had the "diabetes police" watching their every move and reminding them of what to do.

I remember that time of life well. It was during those young adult years that I was diagnosed with T1D. I still feel that T1D stole my college experience. I didn't live a typical college life because of the newness of disease and the fear I harbored. Most stunning though are my memories of both feeling alone and wondering what impact T1D would have on the rest of my life. Like most young people, I was concerned with appearance and perception. Some of my dominant thoughts surrounded how others would think of my disease and me.

Science supports this notion. Perceived negative appraisals by peers have been associated with poorer control for people with T1D (Kyngas et al., 1998). This is a testament to the power of relationships and their impact on T1D. The temptation to ignore T1D and blend in with the crowd is significant and we all fall prey to it.

Social support is critical to good outcomes in life with T1D. By that, I mean number outcomes, social outcomes, and quality of life outcomes! Without loving support, we can't achieve all that we are capable of. With loving support, comes optimism—another critical factor in living well with this disease.

Those who believe they can successfully manage their diabetes are found to be less depressed and anxious than those who believe their diabetes control is a matter of chance or fate. People who have an optimistic outlook on life are more likely to report a higher quality of life (Osborn et al, 2010). Optimism tends to be a significant predictor of both physical and psychological wellbeing.

Because of the importance of social support, loving relationships and optimism, and the profound challenges associated with becoming a young adult with T1D, I created a program for young adults called Students With Diabetes. This is now a national organization with chapters across the country, and is meant to be a social opportunity and a connection point for young adults living with T1D.

It is critical that when thinking about youth with T1D we think in the context of where they live—their reality. We then must tailor education, information, guidance, and tools to match that reality. This toolkit is about meeting young adults where they are. It is about talking through transition issues that they want to discuss. This is meant to be real, raw, and relatable.

Life with T1D is hard. But if you have friends helping you along the way, the tough moments become strength builders and you are richer for the experience in the end.

We hope this book illustrates that you are not alone – we are all in this together.

Nicole Johnson

MOTIVATION

Nicole: Did you know that happy people live longer? Happiness can't protect you from getting ill, but it can urge your healing. It is all about attitude and perspective.

"Happiness does not lengthen the life of seriously ill people, but it does prolong the life of healthy people. Happiness appears to protect against falling ill. One of the mechanisms behind that effect seems to be that chronic unhappiness causes stress, which on its turn reduces immune response" (Veenhoven, 2008).

Those that have been through life with diabetes and have succeeded have something in common—the perspective they choose. It is also about choosing to not let illness steal your drive or your joy. Happiness and perspective can be protective factors of those who live with chronic illness.

Gary Hall, Jr., a 10-time Olympic medalist in swimming and founder of The Race Club could have let T1D stop his Olympic dream. He was diagnosed with T1D leading up to the Summer Olympics in 2000 and made the decision to show the world that life's challenges don't stop you from living. The diagnosis was supposed to end his career as a swimmer, but Gary proved that you can be superhuman—super fast, super strong and super dedicated—all while running on insulin. Gary, now a husband and father of two, suggests that T1D helps him keep perspective in life and teaches him about enduring gratefulness.

Phil Southerland, an accomplished competitive cyclist, is the founder of Team Type 1, the world's first professional cycling team that promotes T1D awareness. Phil is a tireless global ambassador for T1D, a condition he has lived with since he was seven months old. When Phil was a child, his mother was told he would go blind, suffer organ failure, and likely not survive past the age of 25. But Phil and his family had a choice—instead of accepting defeat, they chose to believe that anything is possible. His mother was devoted to making sure Phil understood about possibility, and today he does. A world leader in diabetes who is devoted to making sure children with this disease survive, Phil is a perfect example of turning adversity into strength, or as he says, "going from diabetes to dominance."

Kerri Sparling is a blogger and diabetes advocate, is known for telling it like it is when it comes to life with T1D on her blog: Sixuntilme. Diagnosed at six years old, today Kerri still struggles diabetes—but does so with hope and an attitude of expectation. She has seen that odds can be beaten. Married and blazing a trail in diabetes social media, Kerri forges ahead to make sure no one feels the loneliness she once felt. Kerri helped author JDRF's Pregnancy toolkit.

Ethan Lewis is a T1D and an entrepreneur. He saw a problem in diabetes and decided to use his business smarts to fix it. Today, Ethan's products, LEVEL, are in use across the country. He embodies the "can do" spirit and refuses to accept "no" for an answer by following his gut to make life with T1D better.

Martin Wood has lived with T1D for more than 30 years is and is a medical librarian as well as a successful diabetes blogger. He uses diabeticallyspeaking.com to share his life with T1D in a positive, emotional, and often humorous, way. Martin's mission is to make sure people with diabetes have a voice and a friend.

Hope, devotion, perseverance, attitude and guts are the ingredients that make up these successful lives with diabetes. These commodities are not hard to come by. They start with a willingness as they weave toward choices and end with an attitude of happiness and enduring gratefulness. Each of the featured people made a choice to fight T1D. They wanted something bigger in their lives. They wanted to prove a point. I bet you can relate. We all encounter a lot of decision points in young adulthood. I too had them. The important thing to remember is that decisions are opportunities and they need not overwhelm.

I was diagnosed with T1D when I was 19 years old. I was in the middle of such a remarkable discovery phase of life, and T1D seemed to come in and steal my potential. Thankfully I realized life was meant to be lived, not feared. As you know, I went on to graduate from college, have a career in journalism, win the Miss America pageant in 1999, and become a mother... all despite being told those dreams were impossible. Living requires risk. It requires creativity. It also requires hopefulness.

You too can see incredible things happen in your life with T1D. You can achieve, you can perform, you can create, you can shout out. It is all up to you. To help you find your voice, and because we are all motivated differently, I asked Gary Hall, Jr., Kerri Sparling, Ethan Lewis, and Martin Wood a few questions about how they live with T1D. You might find their answers interesting... I did.

Gary Hall, Jr.

How do you give back to the T1D community?
I serve on the Government Relations Committee for JDRF and act as a Blue Circle ambassador for the International Diabetes Federation. I also serve on the Sanford Children's International Board, building children's hospitals in underserved communities. I'm proud of my association with these influential organizations and their commitment to address the overwhelming demands of diabetes.

Who are your role models/inspirations when it comes to living with T1D?
I have been impressed with Mary Tyler Moore. Today there are more and more role models doing incredible things, folks that have diabetes and haven't allowed the disease to interfere with their ambitious goals and a healthy life. Mary Tyler Moore, however, was lending her time and celebrity to a great cause before there was any national or international organization to address the needs of people with diabetes in a meaningful way.

Who do you turn to when you need help with a diabetes emergency?
My wife, Elizabeth.

How do you deal with people who make assumptions about your diabetes?
Karate.

How do you explain T1D to your friends?

In oversimplified terms, I have a broken pancreas.

What is your funniest experience with diabetes?

I always felt strange about pulling out a syringe, drawing up insulin, and injecting on the pool deck right before a swimming race. In a time when doping in sports is such a problem, the act of administering insulin drew some attention and arched some eyebrows. Especially when I would pantomime my Incredible Hulk impersonation immediately after injecting.

Do you ever feel like you can't handle T1D and how do you get past that mindset?

There are times that I hate T1D and don't want to deal with it. You get to the awards podium of the Olympic Games by getting out of bed in the morning on the days you don't feel like getting out of bed in the morning. Sometimes it's as simple as strapping on your shoes, or testing your blood sugar—doing something when you don't feel like doing it. All of us have those days that we don't feel like dealing with diabetes.

What are positive things that have resulted from your life with T1D?

I've taken up a fight against something worth fighting. There are a lot of good people in the fight against diabetes and I've enjoyed meeting many of them.

What is your advice for young adults living with T1D?

Take care of your T1D and go live life. It doesn't take gold medals at the Olympics to inspire others. If you take care of your T1D and live the life you want you'll one day realize that you've inspired someone else to do the same. That's worth doing, better than winning medals.

Kerri Sparling (www.sixuntilme.com)

How do you give back to the T1D community?

Growing up, my diabetes community was limited to where my mom's car could take me and whom I met at diabetes camp. I'm so, so grateful that the diabetes community has expanded to the online space, giving me 24/7 access to people who really get it. I try to give back to this inspirational community by being an honest and passionate advocate for type 1 diabetes, telling our collective stories, and hopefully showing people that there truly is life after diagnosis.

Who are your role models/inspirations when it comes to living with T1D?

Recently, I attended a meeting of the Joslin 50 Year Medalists, which included people who had been living with type 1 diabetes for at least fifty years. Some had over seven decades of diabetes under their belt. These people are my heroes. They were diagnosed in a time when T1D was misunderstood and poorly treated, and they are still thriving. Their tenacity, passion, and sense of humor both humbles and inspires me. I want to be a Joslin Medalist when I "grow up."

Who do you turn to when you need help with a diabetes emergency?

I turn to my husband when diabetes gets tough, both emotionally and physically. He is the live-in part of my diabetes care team, and his support is tireless, patient, and empathetic.

How do you deal with people who make assumptions about your diabetes?

People who make assumptions are uneducated, and therefore, they need a little Diabetes 101. When assumptions are made or incorrect information is spread, I feel that it's my duty as an advocate for diabetes to set the record straight, as politely and firmly as I can. Diabetes may not have a cure, but ignorance thankfully does.

How do you explain T1D to your friends?

I explain T1D as something that doesn't define me, but helps to explain me. T1D isn't the core of who I am, and it isn't the most important aspect of my life. It's just something I deal with every day, and my friends have always been supportive of my quest for good health because they know I'm more than T1D.

What is your funniest experience with T1D?

I felt pretty bad the morning that my husband woke up with a test strip stuck to his face. Bad, but I still laughed at him before gently picking it off his cheek.

Do you ever feel like you can't handle T1D and how do you get past that mindset?

Diabetes isn't easy. Burnout, anxiety, and depression often are side projects of this chronic illness. It can be overwhelming, managing a disease so intensely every day, knowing you have to wake up and do it all again tomorrow. But that's part of what inspires me to work through moments of burnout, as well. Knowing that I have another chance to try tomorrow makes today's troubles seem a little more manageable, and gives me that inspiration to try.

What are positive things that have resulted from your life with T1D?

When you're diagnosed with a chronic illness, people like to tell you what you CAN'T do. I love when they tell me that I can't do something. Their nay-saying lights a fire under me to show people that I CAN do anything. I'm a strong, confident person, and I feel that diabetes has contributed to that sense of "I'm capable of anything."

What is your advice for young adults living with T1D?

Your numbers don't define you. Your disease doesn't define you. You are still you, with or without T1D. Don't let it make you feel like it owns you. You are in control, even in those moments when you feel you're not. You can do this.

Ethan Lewis

How do you give back to the diabetes community?

I have been fortunate enough to launch Level Foods, a brand dedicated to providing innovative diabetes products that are ultra-affordable and help make managing T1D easier.

Who are your role models/inspirations when it comes to living with T1D?

Over the years I have had the honor of getting to know several people who have had T1D for many years. These are peers, mentors, and role models who I am lucky enough to call friends. They continue to inspire me to take better control of my diabetes to hopefully enjoy the success they've had in giving back to the diabetes community.

How do you deal with people who make assumptions about your diabetes?

People often make assumptions and comments to me that relate to society's misperceptions about what people with diabetes are supposed to look like, eat and do. As frustrating as this is, I always remind myself that these situations are great opportunities to educate the person about diabetes--to help them understand it better.

How do you explain T1D to your friends?

When explaining T1D to those around me, I often relate it to having to take a pill every day. Although managing T1D is much more complicated than taking a pill, both become part of the day. Having lived with T1D for a long time, I don't find managing it to be a hassle, as it is one more responsibility to take care of every day.

Do you ever feel like you can't handle T1D and how do you get past that mindset?

No. I realized long ago that I'm the only person that can manage my T1D! Never let T1D get the best of you... always get the best of T1D!

What are positive things that have resulted from your life with T1D?

Living with T1D has truly been a gift for me. It has given me a positive outlook and a sense of professional urgency to do more at a younger age. This started when I started my first business when I was 16, only to later start Level Foods – a national diabetes brand focused on improving the lives of those living with T1D.

What is your advice for young adults living with T1D?

In order to be successful at anything in life, you need to manage your T1D successfully. This means testing, taking your meds, exercising, and eating healthy. Although it sounds like a lot, these are the simple ABC's of achieving good blood sugar control. Once you become comfortable with your T1D, let it inspire you and drive you to achieve more. Harness a positive outlook and set out to do whatever you want in life – with T1D!

Martin Wood (www.diabeticallyspeaking.com)

How do you give back to the diabetes community?

Share your life story, including your successes and failures, so that other people with T1D can know that they are not alone. The best thing that you can give back to the diabetes community is yourself.

Who are your role models/inspirations when it comes to living with T1D?

I'm inspired by people with T1D, who share the same T1D experiences that I do, and don't let it hold them back from accomplishing amazing things.

Who do you turn to when you need help with a diabetes emergency?

I accept that the responsibility of my T1D falls largely on my own shoulders. Still, no matter how well you manage your T1D, a low blood sugar can happen when you least expect it. Always be prepared, and make sure that you have something nearby to treat a low blood sugar at all times.

How do you deal with people who make assumptions about your diabetes?

Type 1 diabetes is easy to misunderstand when you don't live with it every day. When people make assumptions, take the opportunity to educate them. Where your T1D may vary from one person to the next, so may someone's understanding of how you manage it.

How do you explain T1D to your friends?

I have type 1 diabetes. I can eat and do anything that anyone else can. I simply have to do more math than a person without T1D. I wear an insulin pump to help me manage my T1D. Because my body does not make insulin, I have to consider my blood glucose, carbohydrate intake, and activity levels to make a decision about how much insulin my body needs, with the aim of not giving myself too much or not enough. Where a normal body does this automatically, I have to make these decisions manually, all day, every day, and dose accordingly.

What is your funniest experience with T1D?
I find something to laugh about with T1D every single day. If you can laugh about it, you can prosper with it.

Do you ever feel like you can't handle T1D and how do you get past that mindset?
When I am overwhelmed with my T1D, I reach out to friends in the diabetes community, both online and offline. There is always someone out there who can relate to exactly what you are feeling, and remind you that you can do this, and that you're not alone T1D is a disease that is best managed within a community. No one should ever feel alone with T1D.

What are positive things that have resulted from your life with T1D?
Type 1 diabetes is the best thing that has ever happened to me. I am more aware because of it, I am healthier because of it, and I have met some of the most amazing people on the planet that I would never have had the opportunity to meet without it. In so many ways, T1D has made me who I am. As many times as I've wished I didn't have to deal with it, I am also thankful for it every single day.

Nicole: For me, motivation often comes in the form of challenges. Hearing that I can't or shouldn't do something always makes me want to test limits and prove people wrong. That is just my nature. What is your internal motivator? Finding what motivates you and what causes the fire to rise within you, is part of the secret to happiness. When you are motivated, when you feel challenged and when you feel victorious, you feel happy.

This all happened for me on the national stage during the Miss America competition. In my five years of participation with T1D, everywhere I turned someone was telling me my goal was impossible. I heard time and time again that women with T1D weren't supposed to do things like compete in Miss America. I also heard that I wasn't perfect and therefore wouldn't win. There is some truth here. I am not perfect, but that is precisely why I succeeded. Embracing our challenges and using them to become stronger, to work harder and to be better is the definition of beauty. That became my secret of success. Type 1 diabetes became my greatest companion. Diabetes pushed me and for that I am grateful.

There are plenty of challenges in all of our lives. Transitioning from being a young person with T1D to a young adult is anything but easy. There is so much to consider! The following pages and chapters will hopefully take some of the guesswork out of the transition experience. But more importantly, the next pages will encourage you and show you that you are not alone. Possibility awaits — reach out and grab it!

ON YOUR OWN

Nicole: Going away to college or leaving the family home is a difficult process for anyone. Add T1D to the mix and there are levels of emotions and concerns that are magnified for both the young person and the caregivers. There are also plenty of pitfalls to avoid when it comes to T1D management.

Amanda Mezer faced plenty of questions when she started thinking about going away to college. Her decision-making was anything but a walk in the park.

> *Going Away to College*
> *By: Amanda Mezer*
>
> *When I made the decision on where I would go to college, it was met with mixed reactions. At that point, none of my friends with T1D had gone away from home, so there were few people around who could give me good advice about adventuring and learning to be truly independent. I felt ready to face the challenge, but also nervous. My support team always reinforced the saying that "diabetes should not stop you" from doing anything you want to do, including going to college.*

So, I did it. I moved out of state to college and it was definitely scary, but I learned so much and am so much better for it. I did have a few nights with insulin pump failures/or infusion site failures, but I learned to manage them. In a dorm, there is always someone awake at three in the morning! When I would wake up with a high blood sugar, typically one of my friends would keep me company until my blood sugar came down and I could go back to sleep.

One time, my pump site got pulled and I did not know it. That night, my best friend sat with me for over an hour. She talked to my mom on the phone and said she would call her back if I had a severe problem that night, because my blood sugar was over 500 and I was really sick. She was an incredible support! That night, I knew I had found a true, lifelong friend.

I think the best gift is when friends understand when to ask and when to not ask about T1D. This requires a little education and patience on our part as we help them learn how to react to our disease. My friends have helped me when I have been in times of need, but also do not treat me differently. My best friend does not say much about my T1D unless I look starry-eyed or pale. In those moments, she simply asks if I am okay.

Nothing about being away from home for college is easy, but I have no regrets. I would recommend that anyone who can, go away to college. I am learning how to live on my own while still feeling the protection of having friends close by and a health center on campus.

I have learned that communication with roommates, hall mates, and friends is incredibly important. There are some things about T1D that may not be understood and some of the mechanics of living with the condition may need to be explained. For instance, there are times when

> *it is important to have the privacy to change insulin pump sites. That could be misunderstood and blown out of proportion if not communicated about. Also, it is important to plan for a place to securely store insulin supplies. A little planning will go a long way to making the college experience positive and the transition to independence a little easier.*

Nicole: Amanda gives a great perspective of living with T1D and making the decision to go to college. College is not for everyone and there are loads of different decisions that need to be made in the process of becoming independent. What is right for one person may not be right for another person. It is an individual and very personal decision.

Here are some important things to consider:
- Do you know how to manage your own T1D?
- Do you know how to order your own T1D supplies?
- Are you confident with emergency planning?
- Does your college have a good health service center?
- Does your college have a support network available to you?
- Are you able to communicate about T1D to those that live with and around you?
- Does your roommate understand T1D?
- Will your class or work schedule be amenable to your T1D routine?
- Is there a health team that you trust nearby?
- How do you cope with bullying or those that don't understand T1D?
- Do you get homesick?
- Does your college have a support network like Students with Diabetes?

There is no easy or standard answer when considering moving away from home. The best advice is for you to talk with those you consider your closest confidants and advisors about your decision making. Those advisors could include parents, family members, health professionals, school guidance professionals, teachers, ministers, or friends. Although this is an emotionally charged time, seeking out individuals that can help you weigh the options and develop pro/con guide lists is a good strategy.

Becoming Independent and Managing T1D

Nicole: "Congratulations! You are an adult." At times, becoming an adult is scary. There isn't a guidebook that walks you through what should and shouldn't change. It is daunting to think of the responsibility you acquire in this transition phase. And that responsibility is magnified when you think about T1D and independence. Remember, this shift is hard for both you and your parents. They don't have a guide on how to help you become independent, so you are both in uncharted territory. Be patient with yourself and your family. That is the biggest advice I can give. That will also be the most difficult advice to follow. I know you crave independent living. I did too. Just try to go slow. Independence doesn't happen all at once, it is a process, as you will see in the stories below.

On My Own

By: Paige Wagner

I was diagnosed with T1D when I was five years old, so it should not be surprising that my parents have been heavily involved in my diabetes management over the years. My mother in particular has always been there, trying to shoulder the burden alongside me as much as possible. I have been gently encouraged to take on independence through the years. I started preparing and delivering all of my own injections when I was seven years old. My mom and nutritionists taught me how to cook a balanced meal. And even though it annoyed me, my parents did a good job making blood-sugar tests part of my daily routine. They molded me into a well-managed young woman, but I'm still not completely

---

independent. I'm 21 years old and just graduated from college. I've been an eight-hour drive away from my parents for three years, but they still help me with medical bills whenever they can. I'd be foolish to refuse assistance from the people who love me, but I also know that relying on them forever is not fair.

Parents aren't superhuman. The older I get, the more similarities I see between my parents and other adults, like myself. We both work hard to make ends meet and it costs a lot of money, time, and energy to do that. My parents have been carrying more than their fair share of T1D burden through the years and I recognize that it's finally time to take that responsibility off their plate.

The path to T1D independence is gradual. For me it has involved building relationships with caring friends who have my back. I live with my boyfriend who is there for me when we're at home and I have a local group of diabetic peers through Students with Diabetes. My T1D friends are a constant reminder that I'm not alone and that managing T1Ds is doable. When I am lost and feel like ignoring my health, talking to Students with Diabetes friend helps me get back to reality.

My parents just want to see me succeed and I want to make them proud. Separating from them doesn't mean becoming isolated, it means finding a new source of strength.

Nicole: Next, Amanda shares her experience of launching into adulthood and learning how to communicate about diabetes as an adult. This is never an easy process and I commend Amana for working through a hard time. It is not something that happens easily. Take it slow and one step at a time. Do not be afraid to reach out for help. Always remember, you are not alone.

On My Own

By: Amanda Mezer

Until I was 18 years old, I had loving parents that helped me with my 24/7 job, also known as T1D. I was diagnosed at age six, so slowly over the years I had been learning how to take care of my T1D on my own. However, leaving for school was completely different. I could depend on them being nearby if something horrible happened or I needed any help. I am not afraid to ask for help, but I want to deal with my disease myself. Being three states away from parents and my doctors was something I had to get used to, but I would not have changed it for anything. College is a bubble world in many ways, so I did have a health center on campus that could help me in an extreme emergency. However, I think being not down the street from my parents was helpful in getting my independence.

However, every phone conversation with my mother would be "how's your blood sugar?" or "when was the last time you tested?" or "what is it right now?" within the first few seconds of the phone call. So she was still there for me.

Being in high school, I would want to fight my parents about what I was eating. In college, it became clearer that the choices of what I ate were mine, because I had no one telling me not to eat this or that. Now, I would eat the food and feel the ramifications of the high blood sugar, which soon made me avoid those foods, or in some cases learn how to bolus for them. Eating the worst food in the world would not harm anyone but myself.

Of the people I knew with T1D, many of them had left college if they had gone away from home or they ended up transferring. I was not going to let that happen to me. I wanted to be independent and not let my T1D stop me from going away to school. I wanted to show and encourage other people to go away from home instead of staying near their parents. There were many precautions and safety nets we set in place before I left. I found a second endocrinologist in North Carolina, which was very helpful when I became sick several times. I also met with the health center and set up communication with them, in case I was sick or had a blood-sugar problem.

Type 1 diabetes is not a one-person job, but something that friends, family, and medical professionals help me with. I don't think that leaving home necessarily means giving up parental support. However, it means more responsibility and it also can mean more safety nets. Instead of relying on just a few people at home, in college I had to allow many different people help me.

The nights with an extremely high or low blood sugar were the ones that I realized the help my parents had provided me at home was the most valuable. I would have to now sit up, set alarms, and watch TV to keep me awake until my blood sugar came down to a safe range or came up to a safe range. My mom would still be there on the phone, but what happened if I passed out? I had to be aware of what I needed to do and ask for help sooner than I would when I was home and I had parents that would assist in emergencies.

I found several ways that would help me with being an independent person and successfully manage my diabetes away at school. I had been using a continuous glucose monitor since I was about 15 years old. In college, I used it more habitually to catch the highs and lows. I also had to be more open about my T1D. I was always comfortable telling people, but I had to make sure the RA was aware. Additionally, the health center had to know what my preferences were in an emergency. I also made sure that the people who lived around me knew, in case I needed someone's assistance. My professors knew about my T1D, in case I had a problem in class or missed a class because of the disease. I also made sure that I was eating food that would not cause me more problems than needed. I made careful selections at the cafeteria and also made a lot of food in my room. Sophomore year and on, I requested that I live with a kitchen so I could accommodate those needs.

Fourth, I planned ahead. Instead of changing my site right before bed because I was about to run out of insulin, I would change it in the morning or afternoon so I had time to make sure I had a good site before I went to bed. I also made sure I had plenty of supplies—sites, insulin, reservoirs, insulin pens, and test strips.

With these basic adjustments I was able to make a successful time out of my college career.

Nicole: Independence is about accepting responsibility. There are many choices to be made. Those who have the most success realize that they need others in the process of living, and they then surround themselves with positive people. Successful people are also accountable to mentors, and they constantly strive for self-improvement—they are never satisfied. Both Amanda and Paige have found that relationships make all the difference in their diabetes and their lives as young adults.

As we think about the process of becoming independent and launching our adult lives, many questions flood our minds. First, it is a scary process and it is okay to feel apprehensive about it. Remember though, education empowers. This toolkit is meant to give you practical tools to ease the transition and answer questions from people who have been in your shoes.

In the next few sections, you are going to hear from health professionals, young adults, and a little more from me. The topics we are touching on were selected by other people with T1D between the ages of 16-30. This is not an exhaustive list and if there is something that we didn't cover, please talk to your healthcare team.

LIVING POSITIVELY

By: Emily Shaffer-Hudkins, Ph.D.

As you consider your own perspective on life with diabetes, it is important to know how much the way you think really influences your health and how you use your mind can actually be a tool in your diabetes care.

The degrees to which we live and think positively have well-established links to health. A focus on strengths, resiliency, and the good aspects of life are all part of positive psychology, an important set of factors to learn about and develop in living with a chronic illness. The positive psychology movement began to take root with Dr. Martin Seligman during his term as president of the American Psychological Association in 1998. This type of psychology focuses on positive change, benefits, and wellness, rather than problems or illness. Those leading the positive psychology movement strive to define mental *health* not only as the absence of problems (anxiety, depression, etc.) but also as the presence of positive development. It has been noted positive psychologists seek "to find and nurture genius and talent", and "to make normal life more fulfilling." (Compton, 2005).

Important elements in positive psychology include subjective well-being, resilience, self-efficacy and hope or optimism. These are incredibly relevant topics for young adults living with diabetes.

Subjective Well-Being

Subjective well-being is often described as a person's evaluations of his or her own life. These evaluations include emotional reactions to events, as well as judgments of satisfaction and fulfillment. Subjective well-being differs from other measures of a good life, such as number of friends or salary, in that every person essentially has the right to decide whether his or her life is valuable and filled with a degree of happiness.

How we view ourselves has a lot to do with our transition from dependence to independence. Success in this and all other areas is impacted by a person's belief in what is and is not possible. In fact, research shows that high life satisfaction is a protective factor against mental health problems, and fosters a greater productivity level in society and more positive relationships with others. This is important to T1Ds since depressive symptoms are common for those living with chronic disease.

A person's satisfaction with life and the degree to which he or she experiences frequent positive emotions is linked to better health and functioning. Yet these positive feelings can be difficult to maintain in the face of life's challenges. Another element of positive psychology, termed resilience, examines how individuals are able to successfully adapt in the context of significant adversity or risk. Researchers have determined that the ability to 'bounce back' and thrive through and after adversity is not so much an individual personality trait, but rather a process that is most successful with the presence of certain 'protective factors' in a person's life.

Some of those protective factors are:

- Connections to positive role models
- Self-worth and self-efficacy
- Hope and meaningfulness of life
- Attractiveness to others (in personality or appearance)
- Talents valued by self and others
- Faith and religious affiliations
- Socioeconomic advantages
- Good schools
- Opportunities to learn or qualify for advancement in society

Self-Efficacy

Self-efficacy focuses on a person's belief in their ability to produce desired effects by their own actions. It is how willing individuals are to persist in the face of obstacles and challenges. Self-efficacy beliefs tend to develop over time and through experience. Overall, the most Self-efficacy focuses on a person's belief in their ability to produce influential factor in determining our self-efficacy is past experience and our successes or failures.

What makes self-efficacy such an important element in our lives is that it is a very good predictor of our future behavior (Bandura, 1997). People are more inclined to engage in a behavior or immerse themselves in a situation in which they feel confident. Conversely, people tend to avoid situations in which they doubt their capabilities. Self-efficacy beliefs are strongly linked to how we manage our physical health. Whether or not we decide to adhere to a dietary plan, follow an exercise regimen, or stop smoking are all determined, in part, by our belief of whether that change is possible for us to start and sustain even when things get tough.

Optimism

Optimism relates to the way that we think about experiences. Optimistic thinking has been defined as perceiving good experiences to be attributed to one's own personal characteristics. For example, you got a good grade on a test because you are smart and you studied hard. Or, the person you like asked you out on a date because you are fun to be around. Conversely, a pessimistic thinker attributes good experiences to chance or to things around them rather than personal traits. So, that good test grade was just luck or that request for a date was because the person feels bad not asking you out. The way we perceive the situations, be it successes or failures, in our daily life is directly linked to our physical health. In fact, numerous research studies have shown a relationship between optimism and increased immune function, pain, and increased risk for chronic illness (Rasmussen, Scheier, & Greenhouse, 2009).

Hope, a topic closely related to optimism, has been conceptualized by Charles R. Snyder, one of the founders of positive psychology, as an individual's personal beliefs about his or her capabilities and pathways to achieving important goals. In order to feel truly hopeful about the future, a person must first believe that they can effectively strive for and attain their goals. They hold firm to the belief "I am not going to be stopped." Second, a person must feel confident that they can generate workable routes or paths to attaining their goals. In other words, a person with continued hope or optimism believes that they can get out of jam, overcome barriers, and knows of many alternative ways to attain their personal goals through many alternative ways. They hold firm to the belief "I'll find a way to get this done".

The theory on hope emphasizes the power that is in each of us to self-direct. If we believe we can, we most likely will. Our minds, our goals, and our hearts are powerful and in times of transition the value of self-talk and self-belief cannot be underestimated.

What Determines Happiness?

Happiness is determined by factors across three categories, including a genetic set point, intentional activity, and life circumstances (Lyubomirsky, 2007).

- **Set Point**. Set point is the largest factor contributing to our happiness; it is the expected value of happiness within a person's genetically pre-determined range. Approximately 50 percent of our happiness is linked to our genetics. We all have a range of ability to be happy based on what we're born with. Imagine a ruler and pretend that people can be happy on a scale of 1-6. Some people's ranges are naturally high, so even when they are at their lowest happy level, they may seem a lot happier than other people. In that case, their range could be 4-6. However, some people's ranges are lower, so they don't seem happy that often. They may have a range of 0-2. A person's set point is the level of happiness they usually have within their range. For example, a person could have a range of 3-5 but are usually at a 4 level of happiness, which remains stable over time. This has been shown by researchers in test-retests over 10 years (Lykken & Tellegen, 1996).

It is a good thing that genetics aren't the only thing that makes up happiness, or else we wouldn't be able to get any happier. Changes in life circumstances and intentional ways of thinking and acting help us to move our level of happiness within our ranges.

- **Circumstances**. Have you ever heard someone say that life is "10 percent circumstance, 90 percent attitude?" This is a common saying that we often hear from adults or others trying to help us see that circumstances aren't everything when it comes to our happiness. Psychology researchers have found that this is actually true! Specifically, circumstances, or incidental but relatively stable facts of an individual's life, account for just 10% of one's life satisfaction. Circumstances include things like age, gender, the region you live in, personal history, and occupational status. Some of these items can potentially change but typically take a great deal of time and effort. In addition, they have the smallest link to feeling happier. Therefore, the key to increasing happiness within our ranges is intentional activity.

- **Intentional activity**; in other words, what you choose to do or think, your attitudes, and your goals. It is the most promising part of what determines happiness because, although requiring some effort, it is the easiest area to enact change. Intentional activities can include changing what you do (behavioral), what you think (cognitive) or working to make life better (volitional). Behavioral activities that one person may use to boost happiness include exercising regularly or being kind to others. Cognitive activities could consist of reframing situations in a positive light or counting ones blessings. Finally, volitional activities may include striving to meet important personal goals or contributing to meaningful causes.

Knowing that nearly half of a person's happiness can be boosted with intentional activities has inspired positive psychologists to begin to develop interventions for doing just this. Interventions shown to increase happiness in adult samples include strategies such as devising a step-wise plan to attain one's goals, investing in social connections, performing 'acts of kindness' (i.e., behaviors that benefit others or makes others happy) and practicing grateful thinking (Emmons & McCullough, 2003; Lyubomirsky, Tkach, & Sheldon, 2004; Sheldon, Kasser, Smith & Share, 2002).

Nicole: Positive psychology is important to young adults with diabetes, because it is a tool we can use to improve our health. As Dr. Shaffer-Hudkins noted, a large portion of health is related to how we believe and see ourselves. Why not capitalize off of that knowledge to take every opportunity to improve our outlook on diabetes and our diabetes outcomes? I practice positive thinking constantly and it is one of my biggest secrets for good health!

TRANSITIONING TO ADULT CARE

By: Brian Knox, M.D.

This is an exciting time in life, with many things changing. You may be moving to a new place, starting a new school, embarking on a career, and lots of other things. Along with the changes that keep your life busy, its important not to forget to plan ahead with your healthcare. Whether you relocate during this part in your life or not; you will likely need to transfer care from pediatric to adult doctors, and take a new role in managing your own health.

How to Transition Your Care

It's important to start thinking about this early. Even before you hit the magical 18th birthday and officially become an adult, you should start handling your health just like an "official" adult. You're practically already one anyways.

During your teenage years, it's important to start keeping track of your own health, much of this you probably are already doing. Know what medical conditions you have (or have had), how you are managing them, and what medical providers are helping you with each. You should also start interacting with those providers more directly. While you do still need a parent to go with you for appointments until you turn 18, you can start making your own appointments, calling in your own medication and supply refills, and talking with your medical providers independently.

As you get closer to adulthood, it's important to know *when* you need to change healthcare providers. Most pediatricians and pediatric specialists will not be able to follow you past 18-21 years old. This time of change varies, so just ask, and ask ahead of time. You aren't the first person to have to transfer to adult care, so they can probably give you great references for adult providers. After you have identified whom you can see as an adult, try to make your first appointment with them, before you are unable to see your existing team. This will help you smoothly transition, and not do so at the last minute. Upon making your appointment with a new provider, you should ask your existing provider to forward your medical records. Think of this ahead of time, because you will need to sign medical record release authorizations before they will be able to do so.

The culture of adult care is a bit different than in pediatric care. Firstly, you will be the person that the visit is directed to. You are certainly welcome to bring your parent (or anyone else important to you) after you turn 18, but this will not be assumed. Your adult healthcare provider will expect you to answer questions directly, the focus is on you! The HIPAA law is a federal law that governs what information your healthcare provider can release about you to anyone else. This includes family members. If you would like for your healthcare team to be able to speak with anyone other than yourself, remember to sign a release at the office to allow them to do so.

Outside of knowing your own health, and identifying a healthcare team, there are a few more things to keep track of. Know your insurance information. Likely you are on a parent's insurance. This can last up until you turn 26 under current laws. If you need to change insurance, remember to update your healthcare team's office, your pharmacy, and your supply company. Know where you will fill medication prescriptions. If you are moving, you will need to have your pharmacy transfer these prescriptions for you before you go. The same goes for your supply company.

What This Means for Me and My T1D

As it relates to transitioning your T1D care, here are a few specifics you should know about:

- Healthcare team: You are likely being followed by a diabetes specialist (pediatric endocrinologist), and probably have a pediatrician as well. You need to transition with both of these providers and find adult care doctors that you feel comfortable with and trust. You may feel like your diabetes specialist takes care of pretty much everything, but you should still have a primary care doctor who can focus on your preventive healthcare outside of diabetes, keep you up-to-date with your vaccines, and be available for sick visits.

- Medications: You will need to get all of your medications transferred to a pharmacy near you if you are moving for work or school. If you are using the same pharmacy, be prepared to take over the duty of calling ahead for refills. You CANNOT be without insulin. Make sure that you give them advance notice so that this does not happen.

- Supplies: The types of supplies that you need may vary.

Everyone with T1D needs blood glucose monitoring supplies. In addition to those, if you are using an insulin pump, you will have infusion supplies to obtain, and you will need to know who can help you if the pump malfunctions. Know who these companies are, how to contact them, and how to order supplies ahead of time and establish a predictable schedule so you are never without your necessary medical supplies and equipment. (If you are using a glucose sensor, you will need the same information for your sensor company as well.)

Managing T1D On Your Own

You are probably well adapted to taking care of your diabetes by now. The following is a checklist to make sure you feel comfortable with various aspects of diabetes management as an independent adult:

- Insulin: Insulin comes in several forms, and depending on the type that you use will have varying times of onset, and duration of action. Some are designed to meet your body's basic (basal) metabolic needs, while others act quickly and help you with high blood sugars and with processing the food you eat. You should have a good working knowledge of which insulin you use, how quickly it works, and when it is done working.

- Delivery: Our lives are not the same and are in a state of constant change! This is particularly true for you as a young adult. Insulin can be given in various forms (vials, pre-filled pens, and pumps). Each method has pro's and con's, but the variety is meant to help you best handle the different demands of life. If you find that your existing method of giving insulin, does not jive well with new routines, please talk with your diabetes team to find out if another method may be better for you at this point in time.

- Checking: Be clear with your healthcare team about how often you are and how often your team feels you should be checking your blood sugar. This may vary based on your body and your circumstances. There is no one size fits all approach here. The diabetes tools you are using will impact how often it is recommended you check your blood sugar. A word of caution, always be prepared to check additionally when driving, feeling ill, drinking alcohol, exercising, etc. It is important to ensure that the amount of diabetes supplies you are getting matches your needs, and the additional checking you may have to do.

- Hypoglycemia: If happens. It feels bad, and if severe can be dangerous. Most of the time you manage this on your own with juice, glucose tabs, glucose gels, etc. When severe, you may not be able to help yourself. Now more than ever, it is important to identify people in your life that you trust to discuss this risk and the development of an action plan. These individuals should know how to check your blood sugar if needed, and how to administer glucagon (not to mention where it is).

- Related care: Your diabetes specialist and your PCP will be interested in keeping you up-to-date with preventive care. To do this you need to be aware of the following:
  - When was my last HbA1c test?
  - When was my last eye screening?
  - When were my feet last examined?
  - When was my blood pressure last checked, and what have my numbers been?

- When was my last cholesterol test?
- When was my last thyroid blood test?
- When was my last celiac screening?

Lifestyle Considerations that Make a Difference

Nutrition

Nutrition obviously makes a big difference in how easy (or not) it is to manage your T1D. As your routine changes, your food habits will too. (Yes folks, this is how the "freshmen 15" happens.) Pay attention to the types of food you are now eating, and how different they may be from your patterns when living with your parent(s).

Eating consistently makes a difference in your diabetes care. Try to maintain a pattern of eating early, eating smaller portions, and eating every 3-4 hours. Healthy protein sources are important to include with each meal and snack as this will help reduce blood sugar variations. (Some examples include: lean meats, fish, string cheese, cottage cheese, almonds, and almond/peanut butter.) If you are having more trouble managing your blood sugar after meals, reach out to your diabetes specialist, or a nutritionist who has experience with T1D.

Safety First

There are a few considerations regarding safety that you should always be thinking about. Anytime you are driving, you should check your blood sugar to ensure you are not low and a danger to yourself and others. Drinking alcoholic beverages of any sort is tricky. When drinking you can experience an increase in your blood sugar followed by an exaggerated decrease in your blood sugar, typically many hours after drinking. You MUST be prepared to check more frequently when drinking, so make sure you have the appropriate amount of diabetes supplies with you.

You should never drink on an empty stomach, having some food while drinking can help prevent major blood sugar crashes. If you are drinking, ideally you should have someone with you who knows that you have T1D and can help you if you get low. To someone at a party who doesn't know any better, a person who is hypoglycemic, may just look "drunk." This is where trouble can creep in.

Stress

Times of change can be stressful... so can managing T1D! If you are feeling stressed or overwhelmed, first know that you are not alone. It's important for you to identify who your support system is, especially if you are in a new environment. While a normal amount of stress during young adulthood if perfectly normal, it can sometimes become severe. If you find yourself experiencing an overwhelming degree of stress or blue mood, never hesitate to reach out to a professional. Warning signs that your stress level or mood might be problematic include:

- Interfering with social activities
- It keeps me from sleeping
- Sleeping too much
- Crying for no reason
- Feeling guilty
- Having thoughts of harming myself or someone else

If you find this to be happening to you, you should contact someone for an evaluation right away. Look for a psychologist, counselor, or therapist who can help evaluate your symptoms and provide the therapy to make you feel better. IF you aren't sure if your symptoms are severe enough to reach out, GO! A mental health check-up is okay, just like getting a yearly physical.

Nicole: As individuals with a chronic condition we can't be careful enough. I love Dr. Knox's comprehensive and real life advice. We as patients have the responsibility to constantly seek the best relationships possible with our health care team. It is important to have a team that you trust. Remember, you need to always feel comfortable asking questions. Don't be too cautious and don't be afraid.

Here are a few sample questions to start your conversation with a valued member of your healthcare team:

1. How can varied schedules affect my diabetes?
2. Can you help me strategize about shift work and diabetes care?
3. The stress of school tends to impact my diabetes. How can I better manage diabetes during stressful times?
4. What new resources are available to help me manage my diabetes?
5. Is there a new glucose meter that I should consider?
6. Am I using my medications effectively to get the best results possible?
7. What should I share with my family or close friends about my diabetes that doesn't feel like over-the-top discloser?
8. What are some cheap, easy foods to incorporate into my diet that will not make my blood sugar go wild?

Health Insurance

Nicole: Health insurance is an important part of the life of any person with diabetes. By purchasing health insurance you are paying a certain amount of money monthly or yearly so that part of your medical expenses will be covered and you will be able to buy medications at a reduced cost. For example, without insurance a person with diabetes can pay over $100 for one vial of insulin and blood glucose test strips can cost over $1 per strip. Insurance is meant to help manage the costs of medical care and protect individuals from financial disaster. (FYI: The average cost of a hospitalization for diabetic ketoacidosis is over $10,000.)

Recently the rules and regulations around health insurance have shifted, and honestly we have not seen all the changes that will occur for people with chronic conditions like diabetes. For now, we know that in the United States it is required to have health insurance. If you do not, you are subject to fines and penalties from the federal government. (Penalties for those without insurance can be up to $600 in the first year and increase in subsequent non-insured years.)

Since you must have health insurance, it is important to know some of the basics. Under the new health care laws, the good news is a person with diabetes cannot be denied health insurance. You have options!

If your parents have private health insurance, recent health care law changes allow you to be covered on your parents' health insurance until you are 26 years old. Young adulthood is the time to explore options though and you need to investigate what is best for your particular circumstances. If you work full or almost full time, you may be eligible for private health insurance through your employer. If you are attending college, you may be eligible for insurance coverage through your school. In these instances you need to communicate with either the Human Resources department or the Student Health Services department at your college. Make sure to thoroughly investigate the diabetes coverage elements within all of these different options. Just like in diabetes care, there is no one-size-fits-all insurance plan.

The insurance landscape is confusing. If you are overwhelmed, you are not alone. I struggle constantly with navigating my insurance coverage and benefits.

To best understand health insurance, you must have knowledge of the insurance language. Here are some common terms you will run into:

- **Premium**: The amount paid for an insurance policy. This can be monthly or yearly depending on your plan.
- **Deductible**: The amount that you must pay out of pocket before the insurance company pays its portion. For example, you might have a $500 deductible per year, before the insurance company will cover any of your health care expenses.
- **Co-payment**: A fixed amount you pay for a covered health care service. For example, you might pay a $25 co-payment for a doctor's visit. A co-payment must be paid each time you receive a service.
- **In-Network Provider**: A health care provider on a list of providers preselected by the insurance company. There are also in-network labs and radiology facilities should you need blood work or X-rays. If you choose an Out-of-Network Provider, your costs will be higher.
- **Prior Authorization**: A certification or authorization that an insurer provides prior to a medical service occurring. Obtaining an authorization means that the insurance company is obligated to pay for the service, assuming it matches what was authorized.
- **Explanation of Benefits**: A document that may be sent by an insurer to a patient explaining what was covered for a medical service, and how the payment amount and the patient responsibility amount were determined. This is an informational document that is sent to you. Make sure to always read and have knowledge of what you are entitled to under your insurance plan.

Prescription drug plans are offered through your health insurance plan.

In the U.S., the patient usually pays a co-payment and the prescription drug insurance pays for part or all of the balance for drugs covered in the formulary of the plan. A formulary is a list of preferred drugs covered by the plan. The plan may have a contract with one insulin company and one meter company making those the least expensive choices for patients on the plan. If you want a different insulin or test strip you will have to pay significantly more for it. Some insurance plans have contracts with mail order pharmacies where it is possible to get a 3 month supply of insulin, test strips, syringes and other supplies. Getting prescriptions by mail order is frequently cheaper than buying insulin monthly. For most mail order prescription plans you can sign up online, but you will need a credit card.

For more information about health insurance, The American Diabetes Association and the American Association of Diabetes Educators have compiled fact sheets about the Health Insurance Marketplace and what it means for individuals with diabetes. These are worth a look! (**http://www.diabeteseducator.org/export/sites/aade/_resources/Adv ocacy/AADE_Affordable_Care_Act_Flyer.pdf**
and
http://main.diabetes.org/dorg/PDFs/Advocacy/Health_Insurance_Protecti ons_Final.pdf)

Be assured, health insurance is difficult for most to understand and process. Remember to take it slowly and talk with your family, human resources representative at your workplace or Student Health Services to help navigate the maze. It is easy to get frustrated. Don't fall prey to that temptation. Your health team members are there to help you. If you openly discuss your concerns with them, they will offer their guidance on how to make the best choices for you.

Help for Those Struggling

If you are having a tough time financially caring for your diabetes, there are some resources that might be able to help. Patient Assistance Programs exist in companies like Eli Lilly, Novo Nordisk, and Sanofi. You can find out more about these programs in the appendix of this book.

Portions of the Health Insurance section were developed with the help of Dr. Dorothy Shulman

YOUR REALITY: YOUR YOUNG ADULT LIFE

Nicole: College living is a challenge no matter how you shake it. Mini-refrigerators, budgets, learning how to cook with a toaster oven, cleaning up after yourself—it is enough to put one into panic just thinking about it. Then you add the T1D element and that can push you over the edge. (You know I am being funny right?)

Type 1 diabetes impacts every element of life. It can be a big giant pain in the neck if you let it, but remember the power of control and management is in your hands. Type 1 diabetes doesn't have to steal away fabulous elements of the young adult experience if you don't want it to.

In the next several pages we are going to talk about real life with T1D in young adulthood. You will see several stories from other young adults and will hear a lot of straight talk from me. If I have learned anything in my years with this disease it is to be honest about diabetes reality, as that allows us the opportunity to pursue our dreams!

Body Image

Nicole: Transitioning to independent living is all about negotiation and learning what everyday choices mean to your life with T1D. For many, weight control is a significant challenge. This is related to many factors including different eating habits, alcohol consumption, irregular eating patterns, heavy carbohydrate meals, biology, and T1D management.

Like many of us, Amanda struggled with maintaining her weight during that first year away from home. Change is tough, and society doesn't do us any favors. Amanda learned she had to implement a plan to get on the right track.

How to Avoid the "Freshman 15" and a High A1c When Eating on Campus!

By: Amanda Mezer

Going away to college is filled with adjustments and learning curves. Food was one of the biggest learning curves during my freshman year.

When I was living on campus, I did not have a car and was dependent on the dining hall or campus eateries for meals. This became a huge frustration, especially since my health depends on nutritional information and sound decision making related to food. The food at the main dining hall where everyone eats was unpredictable—you never knew exactly what you were going to get! Sometimes it was actually good and sometimes not so good. There were no carb counts or anything to judge how to dose the right amount of insulin for the foods throughout the dining facility. I was often directed to nutritional information on websites, but unless you carry your laptop through the food line or know in advance exactly what you are going to eat, the benefit from this information was very limited. Who would look online before they went to

---

the dining hall?

To get you thinking about how to strategize your food patterns in college, here are my top five tricks to avoid pit falls:

1. When drinking coffee, I find that asking for half syrup and adding a sugar substitute to sweeten the coffee helps reduce carbs. It also makes it taste less sweet by not adding as much sugar substitute

2. I eat a low carb snack before dinner so that I will not go completely hungry and will not end up eating a carb-loaded dinner.

3. During the day, I eat lots of small snacks and only eat at the dining hall at breakfast or at night to reduce calories and carbs.

4. I limit myself to one dessert per day.

5. I try to drink water with all of my meals to reduce the added calories and carbs from beverages.

The food at college was different than at home. There were many higher carb foods and even the food that I thought was healthy at home seemed to contain a lot of hidden carbs at school. The salad and fruits were often unreliable. And since I am a vegetarian, I guess you could say many days I was trying to decipher "mystery tofu" instead of "mystery meat." So be prepared when you go away to college to be a detective when heading to the dining hall and watch out for those hidden carbs.

Nicole: Amanda's advice is good. Challenges abound when an individual changes patterns or routines, especially food challenges as Dr. Knox pointed out earlier. There are many other body challenges young adults need to consider when thinking about how to manage diabetes during this transitional time of life. Many young adults become tempted to engage in dangerous behaviors to maintain a body image or shape they desire.

Let me be clear – dangerous binging and purging will not have a beautiful end result. Resist the temptation to manipulate insulin and food behaviors to control your weight. Those who binge and purge wind up with much greater issues and often bigger waistlines in the end. It isn't worth the big picture risks of serious health conditions (liver disease, heart disease, high cholesterol), bad breath, damaged teeth, yeast infections, diabetes complications and hair, skin and nail issues. In short, barfing is not beautiful!

If you find yourself tempted with manipulating insulin or disordered eating, talk to your health professional about ways to get help. You can also reach out to the Diabulemia hotline (a non-profit organization) for support: http://www.diabulimiahelpline.org.

Establishing Routines

Nicole: One of the most difficult things during young adulthood is establishing a routine or predictable schedule. Let's face it, predictability just isn't a reality when you are in college, graduate school or in your early career years. This is a time when you must be creative and vigilant about your diabetes. Late night dinners, fun social events with friends, late shifts, early class, lunch time obligations – it all happens. This is your new normal. Don't fear though, diabetes can fit in here.

The first thing you need to know is that *life gets much easier if you are aggressively managing your diabetes.* This means if you aren't, you should consider using fast-acting insulin, an insulin pump and a glucose sensor. There are costs associated with the use of technology, but the benefits are enormous if you can manage the cost. The use of any one of these tools is worth consideration, they can independently and corporately have a big impact on diabetes management.

While on the topic of aggressive management, you should also **be aware of how much time your diabetes care is going to take** now that you are on your own. The volume of paperwork involved in dealing with insurance, ordering supplies, and making appointments can be maddening. Here is a tip, use the apps available that store passwords and special information. This technique will be a lifesaver for you as you work to place your diabetes orders with online pharmacies and as you manage your bills.

Here is the next challenge to consider... *exercise*. As your obligations and responsibilities grow, it may become more difficult for you to work in exercise time. Plus, as team sports become a memory, you may also need to consider new exercise options.

A great tip here is to rely on your friends. Exercise with others is easier, it is social, and it is engaging. Turn your social time into exercise opportunities by engaging in group fitness, popular activities or challenges, and even diabetes fund-raising events. It is about perspective. If this part of your life is exciting, diabetes management will be easier.

For all of the tips and positive spin here, I must tell you some bad news: challenges are constant. At this point in life you are at the beginning of a long road of improvisation and making the best of circumstances. Things will often not go as planned, but if you have a "glass half full" mentality, things will always be ok. Be prepared and plan ahead and you will have the tools necessary to overcome any obstacle diabetes brings.

For those in college, there are a few things you need to know about storing and organizing your diabetes "stuff" that will make life easier for you in the long run.

Let's start basic: Insulin is a must – and storing insulin properly is always important. Make sure you have a dedicated place (refrigerated) for your insulin. Insulin left at room temperature is only good for about a month, and you don't want expensive insulin to go to waste.

In dorms or apartments, refrigerator space and pantry items must be negotiated in advance with roommates to avoid unnecessary misunderstandings and conflicts. Make sure to have a discussion with your roommates about what food and which items are off limits. Have a safe place for your emergency food and be mindful of your diabetes supplies. I hate to say this, but sometimes medical supplies are tempting for thieves or desperate individuals. Take steps early to ensure that your supplies are always safe and there when you need them. A lockbox is a good idea for some, a locked closet might work for others – decide what is best for you by thinking in advance about any circumstances that might interrupt your diabetes care routine.

While on the topic of food, it is often tough for young adults to make good food choices or to figure out how to cook healthy at a time in life when you might not have access to a bevy of cooking appliances. Here are a few recipes that are young adult tested and approved. Plus, they can all be made in a dorm room or an apartment with limited cooking supplies and skills.

Power Breakfast

Including protein in breakfast is a sure way to ward off cravings mid-morning. It is also great for metabolism. Here is a simple dish that can be made with the help of only a microwave!

Apple Oatmeal with Cottage Cheese
- ½ cup of instant oatmeal

- ½ cup of cottage cheese
- 1 small apple
- 1 tsp cinnamon
- 1 tsp of almond slivers

Directions:

- Combine all ingredients, except almonds, into a bowl and microwave to cook the oatmeal according to directions.
- Reserve the almonds for topping after the oatmeal is cooked.

Lunch on the Go

Protein is important at lunch too. Just like breakfast, protein in your meal will help you feel fuller longer and it is a wise choice when counting carbs and/or calories. Here are a few ideas: Consider turkey roll-ups with cheese, Greek yogurt, Edamame Salad, or another form of light protein in your lunch menu. There are a bunch of these recipes online, but here is one that I like a lot from Mccormick.com.

Edamame and Corn Salad

Salad Ingredients:

- 1 package of frozen shelled edamame
- 3 ears of fresh corn (or 2 cups of canned whole corn)
- 1 medium red bell pepper, chopped
- 4 green onions, sliced
- ¼ cup fresh parsley, chopped
- 1 can of black beans (optional)

Oregano Vinaigrette:

- ¼ cup olive oil
- ¼ cup cider vinegar
- 1 tablespoon oregano leaves

- 1 teaspoon garlic powder
- 1 teaspoon sea salt
- ¼ teaspoon ground pepper

Directions:

- Bring 2 quarts of water to boil. Add edamame and cook until tender. Rinse under cold water.
- For the vinaigrette, mix all ingredients in a large bowl. Toss in edamame, corn, red pepper and green onions.
- Refrigerate for 1 hour before serving.

Dinner Delight

Dinner should always be the leanest meal of the day, heavy on vegetables and complex carbohydrates. In this next recipe, I show you how to cut the carbs in a slider significantly by getting a little creative.

Turkey Sliders

Try turkey instead of ground beef. These sliders are an easy meal. If you have a small or countertop grill, these can be ready in five minutes!

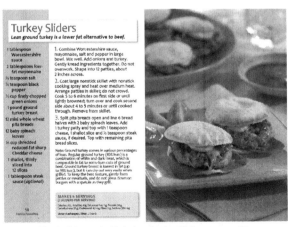

Nicole Johnson's Diabetes Recipe Makeovers, p. 58.
Recipe and Photo © Publications International, Ltd

Food Advice

Nicole: We all become pressed for time in our young adult years. Planning for meals seems to be the last thing on your list, and that is when most people fall victim to the fast food / pizza trap. (I am guilty of this too!) Here is an idea: Consider cooking a few big meals on Sundays and then storing them for ease during the week. When I was in college I would steam veggies on Sunday night for easy lunch and dinners during the early week. I would also keep little bags of fresh veggies ready to take with me for daytime snacking. Low-fat string cheese is a great source of protein for quick snacking during the day, too. Another easy idea is eggs. I often boil several eggs on Sunday nights for quick breakfasts or snacks during the busy week. These are low in carbohydrates, high in protein and great for stabilizing blood sugar.

It is important to also think about alcohol in this regard as well. Alcohol contains a lot of carbs and calories which add up to create that beer gut that none of us wants. Be careful and mindful of the empty calories you consume.

Drugs also have an impact too. Marijuana causes people to get the munchies. Remember, every behavior has consequences and impacts blood sugar levels.

As we consider food, I want to caution that any behavior that is excessive is problematic with diabetes. That means overeating, under eating, purging, withholding insulin, all of these signal big problems for the big picture of seeking a long, healthy life with diabetes. Many young adults are tempted to experiment. Let me be clear, overdoing anything is only a recipe for disaster. If you feel tempted here or are struggling, please reach out and talk to someone about your feelings and thoughts. I promise you are not alone. It will be tough to talk about these kinds of vulnerable topics, but you are worth it and you have the courage to do it!

Alcohol and T1D

Nicole: Risky behavior is strongly associated with young adult experiences. This first brush with independence leads to testing boundaries, trying new things, learning how to manage peer pressure and expectations, and learning how to define yourself.

I have found that the best strategy is to arm yourself with information so that you can then make informed decisions. Dr. Knox shared a little earlier about what alcohol will do to your blood sugar, but there is still more to know. With plenty of information, you can make the choice that is right for you and avoid diabetes disaster. Here are the facts:

Carb Counts in Drinks: Hint - watch the serving sizes		
Drink	**Serving Size**	**Carb Count**
White Wine	5.0 ounces	3.0 - 4.0g
Red Wine	5.0 ounces	3.0 - 4.0g (less if its dry)
Champaign	4.0 ounces	1.0g
Regular Beer	12.0 ounces	13.0g
Light Beer	12.0 ounces	4.5g
Ale	12.0 ounces	5.0g
Guinness	12.0 ounces	10.0g
Appletini	5.0 ounces	8.0g
Margarita	4.0 ounces	7.5g
Pina Colada	4.5 ounces	32.0g
Liqueur (Bacardi Gin Brandy, Rum, Vodka, Whiskey, Tequila)	1.0 ounce	0.0g (it's what you mix with it)

In most states drinking alcohol under the age of 21 is illegal.

What happens when you mix alcohol and T1D?

- Drinking carbohydrates increases blood sugar
- Alcohol makes the liver work harder and causes the liver to "forget" about giving glucagon (stored sugar). Alcohol then tends to decrease blood sugar for 8-12 hours!
- Symptoms of too much alcohol can be similar to low blood sugar symptoms
- Alcohol may cause you to be extra hungry and overeat

How to drink safely with diabetes:

- Always drink on a full stomach, or eat while drinking
- Check your blood sugar, then check and check some more
- Try dosing insulin for fewer carbohydrates than you consume. This may give you a safety net so your blood sugar doesn't drop too low.
- If exercising, try a basal decrease if you wear a pump, or eat extra carbohydrates if you give insulin shots. Exercise and alcohol can be a recipe for low blood-sugar disasters!
- Eat a big snack with plenty of protein and some fat before bed
- Drink slowly and consider alternating non-alcoholic drinks
- Wear your medical ID bracelet, necklace, etc.
- Try to avoid "sugary" mixed drinks, sweet wines, or cordial
- Remember, if you are hung over, you still need to take insulin

The American Diabetes Association suggests that people with diabetes should limit their intake of alcohol to one drink for women and two drinks for men.

A drink is defined as:

12 ounces of regular beer (150 calories)

5 ounces of wine (100 calories)

1.5 ounces of 80-proof distilled spirits (100 calories)

Your best choices:

- Red wine
- Dry or medium-dry white wine
- Dry light beer
- Spirits with "diet" mixers

Nicole: The best advice is to be careful and never drink alone. If you are of age and are going to consume alcohol, do so with friends that know about your T1D and what to do in case you become low. Safety is a priority. Should you feel shy or embarrassed to talk about your T1D with your friends or your date, that is a larger issue. Real friends are supportive of each other, they don't belittle. Remember that.

The Risks of Alcohol

By Paige Wagner

I loved my pediatric endocrinologist. She taught me so much! I thought I knew all I needed to know when it came to managing my T1D... until I entered college and alcohol became a common social activity. I blended into my community of friends and we would go to parties and yes, we would drink. Many pediatric endocrinologists don't address the subject of alcohol with T1Ds and then in adult endocrinology practices it is assumed the T1Ds know how alcohol impacts the body so they never touch on the subject, at least in my experience. I had fun when I went out drinking, but didn't understand why I would feel so terrible towards the end of the night. I just presumed it was a common side effect of consuming alcohol.

I thought I was a fairly responsible person when it came to drinking. I'd always drink water in between servings of alcohol and I'd try to make sure I had food in my stomach before going out, but one night I went to celebrate after a friend's 21st birthday. We drank a wide variety of alcohol and a lot of it. I seemed to be in range at the beginning of the night and that was good enough for me. However, the next morning I woke up feeling like death. I thought I needed to go to the hospital because it hurt to move or think about anything – to basically exist. I was so thirsty, I assumed my blood sugar was high. It was around 300mg/dl when I checked, so I assessed that only water and insulin would help me now.

I proceeded to expel any food that was in my stomach from the night before. I kept drinking water and it made me feel sicker. It wasn't long until I was low, but the change in my blood sugar made no difference in the way I generally felt. I've had bad blood sugar experiences at both high and low levels, but those were quite like this experience.

My boyfriend brought me a smoothie about 3 hours after I woke up. It immediately improved my hangover and brought my blood sugar up to 186mg/dl as well. Still, from the rollercoaster I was on, it hurt to move or think and my horrific hangover wouldn't go away. I was in this terrible state from 10am to about 9pm. Shortly after this experience, I found Students with Diabetes and learned how alcohol impacts the liver and directs all its attention to processing alcohol instead of keeping up with blood-sugar levels. I learned how dangerous alcohol can be for someone with T1D—and while it may be a temporarily fun substance, it's just not worth the risk for me to drink to excess anymore.

I have a lot of friends with T1D who enjoy alcoholic beverages, and if I am with people who understand the risk of drinking with diabetes I feel okay joining in the fun. The silver lining of rarely drinking is that I am not consuming empty calories and my friends appreciate that I am always willing to be the designated driver.

Drugs and T1D

ADVISORY WARNING: Please be advised that the majority of substances listed in this section are illegal.

Nicole: Just like alcohol, drugs can have a serious effect on your diabetes. Research suggests young adults who engage in "regular drug use often have poor diabetic control and more frequent hyperglycemic crises" (Practical Diabetes International, 2005). Therefore, it is smart to know what you're up against if you ever choose to partake. My recommendation is to avoid substances that alter your sensitivity to insulin or to understanding your blood sugar.

Marijuana

When marijuana is used, it acts upon the brain in areas associated with pleasure, memory, thinking, concentrating, sensory and time perception, and coordinated movement. Long-term use of marijuana can be linked to a vast range of mental health issues from increased anxiety to schizophrenia. Short-term use can lead to increased heart rate and respiratory problems. For people with T1D, hyperglycemia can occur as a result of eating large amounts of food due to increased appetite, forgetting to take insulin due to altered perception, increased risk of diabetic ketoacidosis (DKA), and an overall disruption to the normal T1D routine due to overall tiredness and lowered mental ability.

Mo' munchies, mo' problems.

By: Student With Diabetes

In high school, I was a friend to a lot of open-minded people and we liked to partake in things that not everyone was doing. One of the activities we enjoyed was smoking marijuana. Not only did I face punishment and judgment from my mother, but my habitual use caused me to become a little careless with my diabetes care.

My A1c averaged around 8.0-9.0 during that time in my life. When my appetite increased—and it nearly always increased—I would inject a large amount of insulin hoping it would be enough to cover what I might eat. Sometimes my injections were not enough, but sometimes they were too much. It became normal to experience a blood sugar rollercoaster effect as a result of the apathy towards diabetes I felt while high on THC. In regards to school, I was an "A" student in honors classes and well liked by my teachers, I was involved in plenty of extracurricular activities, had a job, went to church, and I exercised daily. I was an involved member of the community! But while every other aspect of my life seemed perfectly in control, the one thing smoking pot diminished was my diabetes management—and that is a very critical part of my life, if you ask me!

In college, there are more people who are smoking and it's very easy to find yourself in situations where marijuana is accessible. Be wise when you make your decisions! Not only do most jobs drug test, but also your health is really on the line if you're at all like me when it comes to smoking. To me, transitioning into independence and college lifestyles can easily take your attention away from diabetes care long before you add drugs into the mix. Once you've found a balance without adding that factor in the mix, I think it's a good time to decide where you stand on substance consumption. Whether it's eliminating drugs completely or just knowing when you can handle the indulgence, the decision is important. Know your body! For me, my health has improved and it just so happens

I no longer use marijuana. I knew I couldn't strike a healthy balance if THC was in the mix.

Hallucinogens

Hallucinogens are known to cause distorted perceptions of reality resulting in an experience that some call a "trip." Theses "trips" often cause fear and panic in the user and with prolonged drug use can lead to more serious paranoia, fear or insanity and disturbing flashbacks. The physical side effects of these types of drugs include increased body temperature, increased heart rate and blood pressure, sleeplessness, and loss of appetite. With diabetes, your awareness of high and low blood sugars will be altered when using these drugs. Because of the paranoia, there is a chance that you might be bothered by the idea of putting anything in or under your skin and you may choose to ignore some elements of diabetes care.

Ecstasy

The use of ecstasy affects mood, aggression, sexual activity, sleep, and sensitivity to pain. The immediate use of the drug can cause increased body temperature, heart rate and blood pressure while long-term or chronic use can affect cognitive reasoning, as well as confusion, depression, sleep problems, cravings, and anxiety. Use of ecstasy also brings on symptoms similar to a low blood sugar. The danger here is if you experience low blood sugar while taking ecstasy, you or those around you may disregard it.

Methamphetamine

Methamphetamine is a stimulant that affects the reward sensors of the brain causing a sense of euphoria in the user. Prolonged meth use damages motor skills and impairs verbal skills. Short-term meth use, even after one use, can cause physical effects such as sleeplessness, hyper activity, decreased appetite, heavy breathing, rapid or irregular heart rate, and increased blood pressure. Long-term use can lead to extreme weight loss and severe mental disorders ranging from anxiety and confusion to paranoia and delusions. Because the drug alters judgment and inhibition, users are more likely to engage in risky and life-threatening behavior. When using meth, those with diabetes may refuse to take treatments out of irrational behavioral and paranoia. For T1Ds, the loss of appetite can result in low blood sugar episodes.

Cocaine

Cocaine is an extremely addictive stimulant that leads to increased energy and reduced fatigue. Cocaine use leads to an excess of dopamine in the brain leading to euphoric sensations for the user. Prolonged users build up intolerance to the drug, which often results in users increasing the amount of drug taken and therefore increasing rick of addiction and risk of adverse psychological and physiological effects. Cocaine abuse constricts blood vessels, dilates pupils, and increases body temperature, heart rate, and blood pressure. It can also cause headaches, gastrointestinal pain, decreased appetite, and increased paranoia. Cocaine users, either short-term or long-term, experience acute cardiovascular or cerebrovascular emergencies that often lead to death. Cocaine also raises blood-glucose levels leading to hyperglycemia.

Heroin

Heroin is an opiate-based drug that enters the brain as morphine and binds to the opioid receptors. Initial use of heroin causes a sense of euphoria that is accompanied by dry mouth, a warm flushing of the skin, heaviness of the extremities, and clouded mental functioning. Just as with cocaine, prolonged use of heroin builds up tolerance in the user, often leading to increased use of the drug and increased risk of addiction. Because some opioid receptors in the brain are located in the brain stem, heroin users are at increased risk for death as a result of suppression of respiration following an overdose. Chronic users may develop collapsed veins, infection of the heart lining and valves, abscesses, and liver or kidney disease. The use of heroin can cause permanent damage to the vital organs and chronic use of heroin often leads to a physical dependence on the drug. As a result, sudden heroin withdrawal can be fatal to the user. Because the immediate use of heroin causes the user to "go on the nod" and experience an alternately wakeful and drowsy state, those with diabetes may be unable to give themselves treatment while taking the drug.

Prescription Drugs

As previously mentioned, many prescription drugs can have adverse effects on your diabetes. The side effects of prescriptions drugs often resemble both high and low blood sugar episodes making it impossible to tell if the user is having an adverse effect to the drug or needs medical attention. Many drugs also impair cognitive response, which could inhibit you from being able to treat your diabetes. You should never take any prescription drugs unless a doctor has prescribed them to you.

The most conclusive evidence about drugs and how they affect diabetes management is that they change your perception and thus are very likely to cause you to forget, ignore, or mismanage your blood sugar levels.

There are many treatment options available for those who are suffering from drug addiction or dependence. If you or someone you love needs counseling to help with addiction, talk to a health professional or call the Addiction Helpline anytime at (888) 299-8125.

Sick Days

Nicole: Let's face it, we all get sick and your young adult years are a time of new experiences and with those come new exposures. It is important to review sick day procedures every time you start a new phase of your life. It is also something you might want to share with those closest to you.

So what should we do when we get sick? This is a question I wrestle with every time I get hit with something as the seasons change. I never can quite remember the "sick day rules," nor do I have the energy to find them at the time. That is why I decided to put this section in here. At least you will be able to flip to this chapter when you start to get the sniffles to just double check your sick day rule memory.

First and foremost, when you are sick you have to check your blood sugar and check it often! Because of the hormones associated with infection, you may need to check every two hours. I know it sounds excessive, but the best rule of thumb is to err on the side "it is better to know than to not know." The Mayo Clinic recommends that people with type 1 diabetes check their blood sugar four times a day when they are sick.

In addition to blood sugar testing, it might also be important to check ketones. Ketones are toxic acids in the bloodstream. You check for ketones by using a ketone strip and dipping it in urine. You can purchase these strips in your local pharmacy. If your blood sugar is over 250mg/dl, then you need to check for ketones. Excessively high blood sugar can lead to ketoacidosis. The Mayo Clinic describes diabetic ketoacidosis (DKA) as a condition where the sugar/carbs ingested can't enter the cells of the body, leading the body to break down fat for energy. This process then deposits ketones into the blood.

This condition can lead to dehydration because the excess sugar passes from your blood to your urine and then triggers a filtering process that pulls large amounts of fluid out of your body.

Ketoacidosis can also cause confusion, difficulty breathing, coma and possibly death. These are the main reasons why people with diabetes must be extra careful when they are sick.

As you have already gathered by the dangers of allowing your blood sugar to get too high, you should not stop your medication when you are ill. In fact, often you will have to increase the amount of insulin to counteract the infection in your body. Your healthcare team will be your guide. Regardless of your food intake, make sure you continue your medication.

My biggest challenge during illness is food. Illness often leaves me unable to or without the desire to eat. And when I want to eat, I often can't figure out what is right for me. In an effort to simplify the sick day drama, here is a short list of some sick day foods adapted from a longer list on the ADA's website **www.diabetes.org**:

- Low fat ice cream (1/2 cup): 10 grams
- Fruit juice bar (3 oz.): 9 grams
- Frozen yogurt (1/2 cup): 15 grams
- Gelatin or Jell-O® sweetened (1/2 cup): 19 grams
- Toast (1 slice): 15 grams
- Soup (1 cup): 15 grams
- Applesauce, unsweetened (1/2 cup): 14 grams

If you have a fever, and you're throwing up or have diarrhea, it is very easy to become dehydrated, which means your body is losing too much fluid. In this instance, take small sips of fluids regularly. Try for a cup of fluid each hour. If you need to raise your blood glucose, try to drink things with about 15 grams of carbohydrate in them. Here are some ideas:

- Apple juice (1/2 cup): 15 grams
- Regular cranberry juice cocktail (1/3 cup): 12 grams
- Ginger ale (1/2 cup): 10 grams
- Sports drink (1 cup): 14 grams

Remember, taking in fluids is key when you are ill. Just beware of climbing blood sugars. Something else that always confuses me is what over-the-counter medications are safe for people with diabetes. According to Drugs.com, there are some data to back up that acetaminophen can cause blood sugars to rise. Talk to your healthcare professional. If you have kidney or liver problems on top of diabetes, you may want to steer clear of this drug.

Drug Ingredients that may affect T1D

Acetaminophen is used in cold and flu medications for minor aches and fevers. Acetaminophen can be toxic to the liver and kidneys. People with diabetes who also have kidney complications should check with their doctor before using acetaminophen.

- Ibuprofen (Advil, Motrin, Nuprin) should be used cautiously by people with liver and kidney problems. It also increases the hypoglycemic effect of insulin and oral diabetes medications.

- Naproxen (Aleve) should not be used for people with severe cardiovascular disease, or kidney or liver problems.

Cough Medicines

- Both Dextromethorphan (Diabe-Tuss, Robitussin, Theraflu, Sucrets, Triaminic, Vicks) and Guaifenesin (Robitussin) are safe for people with diabetes.

Decongestants

- Phenylephrine (Actifed), and pseudoephedrine (Sudafed) are found in both nasal sprays and oral cold medicines. They work by drying the nasal passages. It is possible that they could decrease the effects of insulin or oral diabetes medications.

Antihistimines

- Brompheniramine (Dimetane), chlorpheniramine (Chlor-Trimeton), and doxylamine (Unisom) are used in combination with other active ingredients. These antihistamines do not affect diabetes directly.

Nicole: It is important for us all to be up to speed on what is recommended when we are sick. Being sick is never fun, and it is definitely not the time to have to be surfing the internet to figure out if you should take Tylenol or Advil or Aleve or Motrin. Save yourself the aggravation and get your sick day kit together when you are well. Think of it as your at-home emergency preparedness kit. You might want to include some of the foods listed above and the medications that you and your healthcare team feel are right for you. My kit has all the pain relievers Imodium, Pepto-Bismol tablets, cough drops, nasal spray glucose tablets and cranberry supplements (helps with UTI and yeast infection symptoms). I also keep a bottle of light cranberry juice and Gatorade in my refrigerator, just in case.

Also, make sure to talk to your family members, loved ones or roommates about your sick day kit and about emergency procedures too.

Do they know what to do if you are low and can't respond? Do they know how to help if you are vomiting and unable to eat? Those around you need to be prepared so you can be kept safe and so you feel secure.

If you find yourself in a severe situation that requires hospital attention, you should again be aware of how to be advocate for and protect yourself. Paige will share next about her experience in the hospital with T1D and how she was relied upon as a guide for her care.

T1D in the Hospital
By: Paige Wagner

"If you've ever been to the hospital, you know that it is not a fun place to visit...and it's even worse when you have type 1 diabetes. Very recently, I was rushed to the Emergency Room after severe food poisoning, which led to non-stop vomiting, extreme dehydration, and gastrointestinal bleeding. Being a diabetes veteran of 18 years, I managed to keep an eye on my blood sugar levels while I was passing in and out of consciousness. I take Lantus in the morning, but had not taken any that day (as I was too busy being sick). On an average sick day I'd anticipate lots of high readings—especially without Lantus-- but interestingly, I was coasting in range through all of my illnesses (roughly 80-160mg/dl). It didn't make much sense to me, but it put me at ease that my diabetes likely wasn't the cause of how terrible I felt.

Over my three-day stay I learned that the doctors and nurses taking care of me knew very little about diabetes. Even worse, they knew nothing about MY diabetes. There were miscommunications about when I took my long acting insulin, there were times I had to insist on more rapid acting insulin than had originally been ordered by the overseeing doctor.

There was a nurse who actively argued with me over what needed to be

---

done, but I know what I need so I had the order changed for the proper amount of insulin.

Multiple people on staff would ask things like: "Do you typically run high or low?" and "Do you have your diabetes under control?" We'd been doing blood work every 12 hours, so my HbA1c was right in front of these people!

I was able to manage my blood sugar because I advocated for myself and had people advocate for me while I was in critical condition. If my family and I hadn't been engaged in each aspect of my hospital stay, there's a good possibility they would have kept me in the hospital even longer!

Don't get my wrong; I am grateful for the care I did receive because I got better. Although I wish there was a more complete understanding of diabetes, I have learned to be forgiving when others don't get it like I do. Doctors and nurses will do their best to take care of you, but their best effort will never come close to yours."

Nicole: Remember, you are the expert on your diabetes and your medical history. Make sure to keep records and communicate about your condition with others to ensure that you are staying healthy and safe. Sometimes this means even arguing for yourself and questioning the tactics of others as they seek to help care for you.

Mental Health

Nicole: We all know that Type 1 diabetes affects more than just your physical body. It plays a role in emotions, in moods, in your general outlook on life, and it can affect your mental health. It is important to realize that there isn't shame or isolation in the emotional and psychological challenges related to diabetes. In fact, studies have found that individuals with diabetes are more likely to experience depressive symptoms than those without this condition, often due to the increased burden and responsibility of treatment and the overall impact diabetes has on quality of life (Egede & Ellis, 2010). It is estimated that about 30 percent of those living with a chronic illness like diabetes also experience some mental health difficulties, including depression and anxiety (Li, Ford, Strine, & Mokdad, 2008). The most important thing, as already mentioned by Dr. Knox, is to ask for help when you feel worried or unable to cope. Amanda delves into this topic in a very personal way next. She doesn't give up and you shouldn't either.

Depression with T1D – Now What?
By: Amanda Mezer

The word "depression" has many meanings today. Additionally, there are many types or degrees of clinical depression. What is the difference between your feelings after a death in the family or an illness like pneumonia and the feelings chronic condition of depression? The short answer, I found, is nothing. They feel the same but the difference is the length of time the feelings exist.

In January 2010, I was diagnosed with a chronic major depressive disorder. I associated the down feelings I was having with many life events, including pneumonia, an injured knee, and my grandfather's death. As a second semester freshman in college, there was so much stress being far away from home and more academic work than I ever had before it seemed reasonable to feel blue. I didn't know what I was about to face or the seriousness. I continue to ask myself many questions about the how and why related to my diagnosis. When should I have been concerned that something was wrong? Wasn't I just feeling the emotions of a normally over-stressed college student? What could have been done differently?

The actual feelings and what is written about depression can be far from reality. The feelings are much more intense and painful than anything I had experienced before and what I had read about them. As a young adult, I did not know what to do or where to go. I found that even as I did start reporting symptoms, I was not getting the help I should have gotten. I knew something was wrong, so I took the initiative to go to the counseling center. I did not know what was wrong, but I knew what I was feeling. Later, I found out that the counselor was not taking me seriously and thought I was being overdramatic. As I became sicker and sicker with depression, she continued to ignore me. Finally, the counselor admitted that I needed help.

I talked to many different professionals before I got help. However, that extended period of time made the depression harder to treat. If someone gets help sooner rather than later, there is less difficulty bringing the person back to where they once were, even if they are dealing with a chronic condition.

Depression is a chronic condition, so just like T1D I have to take medicine every day. As long as I exercise, eat healthy, and get enough sleep, I do fine. Many people with T1D have depression and to varying degrees, which is something I did not realize until this experience. If you are feeling down, like I did, talk to someone! Reach out! Be persistent! I got through this horrible experience because of a good medical team and supportive friends and family.

It is important to know that depression, like T1D, is a treatable condition. With the proper diagnosis and treatment, it is manageable. It is also important to know how you are feeling and take action when you think it is necessary. Just as it is easier to treat a high blood sugar of 250 instead of 400, it is easier to treat depression when the symptoms are minor instead of severe. Just like with T1D, you feel better when your blood sugar is under control, you will feel better when your depression is under control. I am living proof!

Emily: Although there are still daily challenges for Amanda, she has learned some key things to help manage her depressive symptoms. What we know is that often a combination of medication and behavioral changes can improve the way a depressed person feels day to day. Understanding the side effects of medication for depression as well as how this may impact diabetes management is very important. When we are feeling sad or depressed, we have a tendency to want to avoid our daily activities and social interactions. Even though it is tough, doing a few enjoyable activities each day, such as going for a walk, calling a supportive friend, or going shopping, can start to improve a depressed mood. Paying attention to your thoughts is also a key part of managing how you feel. Focusing on good events and attributing those to your own personal strengths and characteristics and seeing bad events as temporary and not reflective of you as a person are directly linked to improvement of depressed feelings.

Many people report experiences similar to what Amanda describes when meeting with medical or mental health professionals—there is little talk about how our physical and mental health are related. Although some cultures worldwide have historically placed a lot of emphasis on the mind-body link, only in recent years have those in Western medicine started to focus on the 'whole person'. We now know that how a person feels physically relates to his or her emotional state and day-to-day thoughts. As Amanda emphasized, it is important to manage both your physical as well as your mental health in order to be at your best.

Traveling with T1D

Nicole: In my over 20 years with t1D I have done my fair share of traveling. I once counted over 3 million miles! I am lucky to have only had a few challenges.

There have been plenty of Transportation Security Administration (TSA) moments where I have been frustrated by the lack of understanding about my insulin pump or glucose sensor. Amanda will share more about that in her story later. My real emergencies though, mostly came from lack of preparation. There is an old adage that says you never plan to fail, you just fail to plan. We all always have good intentions, but life happens. When I became a mother, my organization about my diabetes went out the window. I would go on trips where my baby would have triple what she needed, but I would forget all of my T1D supplies.

There have been other times when traveling internationally I have had pump mishaps and I was not able to get a replacement and then was forced to scramble to find the long acting insulin I needed to cover my blood sugars while I was without a pump. But I have learned that it is necessary to have an extensive packing list and to use it for every trip, whether a weekend getaway or an international excursion.

So, here goes a glimpse into traveling with Nicole.
Health checks before you go:
- Family doctor
- Dentist
- Eye doctor
- Diabetes clinic

Vaccinations

Talk with your doctor about where you are headed and any vaccinations that might be needed to protect you and keep your diabetes in good control. Make sure to initiate this visit a few months before you travel. Some vaccinations need multiple doses and require time lapses.

Documentation

Make sure to carry multiples of your important documents. You should have one set of copies with you at all times, another with your family or loved ones at home, and another potentially in your luggage or with your traveling companion. If anything gets lost or stolen, you want to be able to talk to the authorities and get what you need fast! Get a letter (on letterhead) from your health care professional explaining that you have T1D and need to carry medication, glucose testing supplies, etc. Get a prescription letter from your clinic with all the medical items you may need. Medications should be listed with both generic and brand names. Syringes and blood testing items should be listed as well.

First Aid Kit
- Pain killers/aspirin
- Allergy medicine
- Anti-diarrhea medicine
- Motion sickness medicine
- Sunscreen
- Insect repellent
- Wound kit: bandages, antiseptic, and blister treatments

Diabetes Kit

A good rule of thumb is to always carry double what you think you will need in T1D supplies:
- Insulin

- Syringes or pen needles
- Pump supplies
- Batteries
- Glucose meter
- Lancets
- Extra lancing device
- Test strips
- Glucagon kit
- Glucose tablets or gel
- Emergency food

We all know that anything can happen during travel, and as you can imagine with over 16 years of T1D road experience I have had some doozies!

Travel plan

What is a travel plan and how do you create one? I always have some kind of plan regardless of the kind of trip I am on. For instance, I always make sure to know in advance food arrangements during air travel. With this information, I decide what types of snacks to carry on with me. It is also helpful to know how long the plane will be in the air and connection times.

Friends often wonder why I make certain requests when I travel, but it is all based on my travel plan. I try to make sure to always stay in hotels that have 24-hour food service and a fitness center. These are necessities for me to manage my T1D in a wise manner. Remember, that if you are changing time zones, it is important to have constant access to food. Our bodies are often unpredictable in these situations and it is a challenge to adapt our circadian rhythms quickly. If you are traveling internationally, a travel agent can help you with information important to your travel plan. You need to know the closest hospitals to your hotel and how to get medical care should you need it.

Here are a few other things to consider when traveling and creating your travel plan.

Meals

- Take plenty of carbohydrate foods with you. Be prepared for travel delays.
- To be safe, when traveling by air, wait until you see the food to inject medication.
- Carry plenty of glucose/sugary foods in case you feel low. Some airlines do carry a glucagon kit, however, personnel are not usually trained on its use.
- Check your blood glucose regularly. During travel you may find your results will be higher than usual, probably due to sitting for long periods.
- If you suffer from travel sickness take a bottle of juice or soda with you in case you cannot eat.

Typically, I have made several stops prior to boarding the plane. I check my glucose before I get to the gate, I always buy some sort of emergency snack for the plane, I always have a cell phone and charger handy, and I always have my medical identification in plain view. It's very important to plan ahead.

Transporting and Storing Insulin

- Insulin should never be kept in luggage going into the hold of the plane. Often temperatures drop below freezing and there may be pressure changes that could cause damage.

- You can carry insulin in a variety of ways: cool bags, zip lock cases, makeup bags or medical specific containers. The best decision is the one that best suits your lifestyle and your individual needs.
- Because of liquid restrictions during air travel, you may want to avoid ice blocks or ice packs.
- If you are keeping insulin in a backpack, make sure it is protected from direct sun damage. If in the top pockets, double protect the vial.

I often carry two bottles of insulin when I travel. One vial is in my makeup kit and the other is in my purse. I can rely on these bottles and know that there is always a backup. There is also always an emergency syringe with the vials of insulin in case something happens to my pump.

Pumps

If you use a pump, the same rule about being doubly prepared applies. Always have twice as many supplies as you think you will need. When you use a pump, it is also a good idea to carry syringes or an insulin pen just in case. This is particularly helpful when traveling out of the country. Not every country sells the same products. At times, it can be difficult to find specific supplies. Being double prepared can save you a lot of hassle and even a trip to a foreign hospital.

Again, most of your supplies should be carried in your hand luggage. If you are packing some of your extra supplies in checked baggage, consider splitting them up in all of your bags. If you are travelling across a few time zones, remember to change the clock on your pump to the new time zone. It is up to you to decide when you want to change the clock. In my T1D care and travel experiences, it works best for me to change when I board the plane. However, everyone is different.

If you are traveling across many different time zones (four or more), you may want to set a temporary basal rate at your lowest basal rate for the amount of time you will be traveling, and take a bolus dose each time you eat or every two hours depending on your glucose results. You should check your blood sugar more frequently during the time you are traveling and until your blood sugar settles.

Traveling with T1D is possible and can be very enjoyable. Remember to be prepared, develop a travel plan, and anticipate problems before departing. These tips will save you a lot of time and headache during your vacation.

Amanda has also had some interesting travel experiences. Here is her story about traveling with diabetes technology.

Airport Security and Insulin Pumps

By: Amanda Mezer

As a college student with T1D, I find that I am traveling more and more by plane. I'm amazed how often a security person asks me to "take my iPhone or iPod off (which is known to us as insulin pump), but sometimes the conversation goes further or becomes comical or embarrassing.

One time, the security guard sternly said, "Take that off" but once I said it was an insulin pump, he replied in an equally stern manner, "Keep that on!" I have been told by Minimed that I should not go through the newer security machines that look through your clothing because it could harm my pump. When I am told to go through one of these devices, I ask for

---

the pat down instead. Sometimes the security person says, "Oh, it's okay, it won't hurt anything," but I stand up to them and make sure my pump is safe.

However, my most frustrating situation happened when I walked through the regular metal detector and the alarm did not go off, but the security person saw my pump and said that I had to take it off and go back through again. I said, "I can't, it's an..." but he kept interrupting me. I kept attempting to say it was an insulin pump, but he wouldn't listen. He said, "I don't care what it is, take it off!" I soon found out that he was new and was in training. His boss stepped in as I got tears in my eyes and told me I could go through. The boss then explained to the trainee that it was an insulin pump.

Over the years, airport security agents have become more aware of insulin pumps. Surprisingly, at some security points, they have actually asked if it was an insulin pump instead of assuming it was not. I think this is great and I really appreciate that there is an effort being made to make security more comfortable for all of us.

It is important to remember that going through security when you travel can be stressful, but knowing what to expect and what you can do to protect your supplies will make it easier and more pleasant. Communicate with the security agents and relax.

Graduate School

Nicole: Perhaps you are thinking about what is next in your life journey. College was an easy decision, but now you must decide if you feel prepared and ready to begin a career or if you prefer to advance your academic training by continuing on to graduate school.

If you choose to pursue an advanced or professional degree, you will be required to take an advanced level standardized test or professional exam such as the GRE or LSAT. You thought you were finished after the SAT didn't you?!

It is important to note that as with college standardized testing, special accommodations are available for the GRE and other similar graduate education tests. To get these accommodations though, you need to do a little advance planning. If you decide to take the test at the last minute, you may be out of luck. The review process for accommodations requests may take six weeks or more once your request and all required paperwork have been received. Some exams (e.g. GRE) will **not** allow you to register online if you are requesting accommodations as the accommodations request must be approved prior to registering. Other exams (e.g. LSAT) require that you register for the exam before you request accommodations. Be sure to visit the official website for the specific test you need to take in order to ensure you adhere to the all requirements necessary for requesting accommodations.

When registering for your exam, do yourself a favor and schedule your test for the time of day that is best for your blood sugar. Also, if possible, use a private room. Make sure to communicate with the supervisor about your T1D testing and your needs. Stress can make a person with T1D have major blood-sugar swings. When I took the GRE my blood sugar went sky high, which certainly didn't help my score.
Be aware, most testing sites do not allow food or beverages or glucose meters at the regularly scheduled tests.

Here is what ETS says about diabetes and accommodations:
"Test takers with health-related needs may be able to test under standard conditions if ETS determines that only minor adjustments, if

any, to the testing environment are required Test takers who wear an insulin pump do not need to be approved for accommodations unless the pump is especially noisy. In that case, it is recommended that testing take place in a separate room so the noise will not disturb other test takers. Candidates who require food, a beverage or equipment such as glucose testing materials or an inhaler must apply for accommodations also, since a separate room may be necessary."

How to Request Accommodations

To receive accommodations, the test taker may be required to submit documentation identifying the prior 6 months of disease and detailing manifestations of the health condition. If the condition is episodic, expect the testing agency to require documentation that outlines frequency and duration of the test takers current limitations and the need for accommodations.

In identifying the need for accommodations and the presence of a diabetes, it would be advisable for the test taker to provide a letter from a health professional that details the specific diagnosis, a description of current functional limitations, medical information about any restrictions, side effects of prescribed medication and any other possible explanations for functional limitations that impact the ability of the test taker to take standardly administered tests.

At the time of the test, the test taker should be prepared with the accommodations letter from ETS, an additional copy of the accommodations request, an additional copy of the documentation from a health professional, and a copy of the ETS disability policy.

Plan in advance if you choose to seek accommodations. These requests can take up to 6 weeks to review.

Planning ahead is important. Following you'll find contact information to request accommodations. If you need further assistance, visit the student health services office or the human resources group at your place of employment.

Contacting ETS Disability Services Monday–Friday 8:30 a.m. – 4:30 p.m. ET

Phone: 1-866-387-8602 (toll free) from U.S., U.S. Territories* and Canada

Fax: 1-609-771-7165

E-mail: stassd@ets.org

Mail:
ETS
Disability Services
P.O. Box 6054
Princeton, NJ
08541-6054

Nicole: It is important for us to always know our rights and responsibilities with diabetes. I hope you will never have to take action related to your rights, but just in case you have to argue for yourself, remember the best policy is to educate, negotiate and then litigate. Most every situation can be resolved with patience, open conversation and a little knowledge about the Americans with Disabilities Act (ADA). You will learn more about the ADA in the next chapter. ☺

Diabetes in the Workplace

By: Ashley Wingert, MPH

Entering the workforce is quite an adjustment. Maybe you had a part-time job in high school or in college, so you already know where to wear your pump, but preparing for a full-time career introduces new challenges. The extended work hours and responsibilities of a full-time position may not seem like a huge adjustment in theory, but in actuality the stress tends to be greater than anticipated. Working full-time means added responsibilities – and more people depending on you. The reality that this position may lead to a career provides added pressure to impress your superiors and get along well with your co-workers.

Is someone going to complain that I take too many breaks? What if I can't make it into work – what's the proper protocol?

It is important to establish open communication with your superior early so when a need arises, you feel comfortable talking with your boss. You should also consider disclosing your diabetes with your co-workers so there is greater understanding regarding any challenges you may face. If you have a low blood sugar and need to take a lunch break earlier than your scheduled time, it may be easier to convince a co-worker to switch lunch breaks with you if he/she understands your personal situation.

A word of caution though: Don't allow your diabetes to become an easy crutch in the workplace. Constantly complaining about your struggles with diabetes or using diabetes as an excuse to be late for work may both annoy your co-workers and lead them to doubt your abilities.

Moments will certainly occur when diabetes impacts your work performance, but recognize the difference between these moments and the temptation to use diabetes as an excuse.

Conversely, you don't need to have a hero complex. If you're stressed at work because you have a hundred things to do, ignoring a low blood sugar may seem like a good idea because you can deal with it "later", but doing so may compromise your work and your health. Taking care of your diabetes is important because it allows you to perform your best at work. The discipline that accompanies managing diabetes can actually be a benefit to you in the workplace and can be an opportunity for you to impress your superiors.

One thing to keep in mind when choosing a career is that some fields are more stressful and/or physically demanding than others. Working in an Intensive Care Unit at a hospital is vastly different from working as a financial specialist for a large business. Both careers can be stressful and demanding, but for entirely different reasons. When you begin your career, think about how the demands of your job may impact your diabetes so that you can plan accordingly. There is nothing you can't do because of your diabetes – to fulfill your dreams however, it is to your benefit to plan ahead!

What you need to know:
- Diabetes alone can't keep you from job promotions.
- If you share an office refrigerator, label your food.
- Find your "safe place" for diabetes care at the office (it doesn't have to be the bathroom).
- Beware of candy bowls and other office treats.
- Befriend the "Office Mom."
- Always be prepared with extra diabetes supplies at work – in your desk, car, bag, etc.
- If you wear a pump, set the least noisy alarms or reminders.

- Plan your outfits accordingly: don't forget about diabetes gear.

YOUR LEGAL RIGHTS

No matter what people say or try to argue, diabetes, as well as other chronic illnesses, is protected under the American With Disabilities Amendments Act of 2008 (ADA). The ADA prohibits discrimination against people because of their T1D in either the workplace or in places of public accommodation such as colleges or universities.

Americans with Disabilities Amendments Act 2008 (ADA)

The ADA protects qualified individuals:

- who have a physical or mental impairment that substantially limits one or more of a person's major life activities;
- who have a record of such impairment; or
- who are treated as though they have such an impairment

The ADA defines major life activities as, "basic activities that an average person can perform with little or no difficulty, such as eating or caring for oneself, performing manual tasks, seeing, hearing, eating, sleeping, walking, standing, lifting, bending, speaking, breathing, learning, reading, concentrating, thinking, communicating and working." (ADA Amendments at § 4).

Prior to the passage of the ADA, most of the litigation claiming diabetes should not be considered a disability pursuant to the Americans with Disabilities Act of 1990, focused on the argument that a person could manage diabetes with diet, exercise, medication and/or technology in a way that would not substantially, if at all, limit any major life activities. The ADA refutes that argument and further defines a major life activity to include, "... the operation of a major bodily function, including but not limited to, functions of the immune system, normal cell growth, digestive, bowel, bladder, neurological, brain, respiratory, circulatory, endocrine and reproductive functions. (42 U.S.C. § 12102(2)(B)).

For example, T1D becomes a disability pursuant to the ADA when it (1) substantially limits how a person, eats, cares for themselves and or performs manual tasks that an average person can perform with little or no difficulty, (2) causes complications or side effects that substantially limits a major life activity. Even if the T1D is not currently substantially limiting because it's controlled by diet, exercise, medication or technology, the condition is still a disability because it was substantially limiting in the past (i.e. prior to or at diagnosis), and (3) does not substantially affect a person's life activities, but a third-party assumes that it does.

Diabetes and Discrimination (colleges and universities)

All places of public accommodation, including non-religiously controlled colleges and universities that receive federal funds, are subject to the rights and responsibilities outlined in the ADA. In other words, a student cannot be denied admission to a public college or university because of his/her T1D, and the college or university is required to provide qualified students with any and all appropriate academic adjustments to afford any student with diabetes an equal opportunity to participate in the school's program.

It is your responsibility to seek any special modifications, adjustments, services or aids. All requests, including the necessary documentation, should be made to the appropriate dean, program or faculty members. Colleges or universities will not change academic requirements, but are required to approve all reasonable requests to enable a student with diabetes an equal opportunity to meet those requirements. Do not be afraid to ask... it's your right!

For example, the ADA provides that, "Modifications my include changes in the length of time permitted for the completion of degree requirements, substitution of specific courses required for the completion of degree requirements and adaptation of the manner in which specific courses are conducted." (Statement of the Manager's to Accompany S. 3406, The Americans With Disabilities Amendment Act of 2008).

Diabetes and Discrimination (workplace)

The ADA prohibits discrimination in the workplace by private employers with 15 or more employees as well as state and local government employers. The Rehabilitation Act affords the same protections to federal employees and the states have laws that address private companies with less than 15 employees. For the purposes of this section we will focus on the protections guaranteed by the ADA.

When seeking employment, make sure to keep the following list of protections from the ADA in mind.

- You are not required to disclose that you have diabetes, or any other health issue
- If you voluntarily disclose that you have T1D, a prospective employer can ask if you need reasonable accommodations, and if so, what are those accommodations
- An employer cannot rescind a job offer because of your diabetes unless it's determined you cannot do the job without reasonable accommodations or pose a threat to the safety of the other employees

After you have accepted employment remember these are your rights according to the ADA:
- You cannot be terminated because of your diabetes, unless you cannot perform your employment duties without reasonable accommodations or if you pose a threat to the safety of other employees
- If your employer has a legitimate reason to believe that your diabetes is affecting your performance, the employer may ask questions or require you to submit to a medical examination
- Your employer cannot request medical information because of poor performance. Your employer can only request medical information if they have a reasonable belief that your diabetes is causing the poor performance
- Other than performance issues, your employer can ask about your diabetes only if you've requested reasonable accommodations and/or if you are participating in a voluntary wellness program
- If, and only if, it's part of the policies and procedures manual, your employer can ask for a Dr.'s note to justify the use of sick days. Otherwise, they cannot ask.
- An employer cannot disclose you have diabetes to the other employees. They can explain the special accommodations, but

cannot disclose that you have diabetes. It's helpful if all special and reasonable accommodations available to employees be outlined in policy manual.

Examples of reasonable accommodations:
- A private area to test blood sugar, inject insulin, take medication, or use an insulin pump or sensor
- Private place to rest if blood sugar levels go outside the normal range
- Breaks at reasonable intervals throughout the day to test, eat, drink, or take medication
- Time off for treatment, recuperation, or diabetes training
- Modified work schedule or shift change
- The use of stools, glasses, or aids due to complications

An employer is not required to grant all reasonable requests if doing so will cause an undue hardship on the employer. An undue hardship is anything that causes significant difficulty or expense. Testing and managing your diabetes in the workplace is your responsibility. Your employer cannot ask about testing or any other part of your T1D management regimen, unless they have a reasonable belief it's affecting your performance.

Safety on the Job

An employer can ask you about your T1D only it believes that you pose a "direct threat" to yourself or others. For example, an ironworker works at construction sites hoisting iron beams weighing several tons. A rigger on the ground helps him load the beams, and several other workers help him to position them. During a break, the supervisor becomes concerned because the ironworker is sweating and shaking. The employee explains that he has T1D and that his blood sugar has dropped too low. The supervisor may require the ironworker to have a medical exam or submit documentation from his doctor indicating that he can safely perform his job.

Your employer can require you to leave your place of employment and submit to a medical evaluation if it has a reasonable belief that you are unable to perform your job or pose a "direct threat" to others. Any questions must be limited to obtaining that information which is necessary to assess your present ability to perform your job. For example, a telephone repairman had a hypoglycemic episode right before climbing a pole and was unable to do his job. When the repairman explained that he recently had begun a different insulin regime and that his blood-sugar levels occasionally dropped too low, his supervisor sent him home. Given the safety risks associated with the repairman's job, his change in medication, and his hypoglycemic reaction, the employer may ask him to submit to a medical exam or provide medical documentation indicating that he can safely perform his job without posing a direct threat before allowing him to return to work. (www.eeoc.gov)

Service Animals

Another area where your legal rights may come into question is with service animals. Diabetes Alert Dogs are growing in popularity in the Type 1 Diabetes community. In 2010, the Department of Justice published revised regulations implementing the ADA for State and local government services (title II) and public accommodations and commercial facilities (title III) with respect to service animals.

In the law, service animals are defined as dogs that are individually trained to do work or perform tasks for people with disabilities. The work the dog is trained to do must be directly related to the person's disability. A dog that provides emotional support or comfort does not satisfy the definition of service dog.

The ADA provides that service dogs are allowed to accompany people living with diabetes in all areas of a facility where the public is allowed.

There are a few rules though:
1. The service dog must be under control, and
2. The service dog must be housebroken.

What is Acceptable With Service Dogs?
1. Limited inquires are allowed. Business owners and staff can ask:
* if the dog is a service dog and
* what task is the dog trained to do
2. A business owner or staff cannot ask you to leave because of the service dog unless the dog is not under control or housebroken.
3. A service dog must be allowed in places that serve food even if state or local laws prohibit animals on or in the premises.
4. You cannot be isolated from other patrons because of a service dog or served differently in any manner.
5. Staff of a business are not responsible to provide food for the service dog.

For more information about service dogs and your rights visit www.ADA.gov

RELATIONSHIPS AND DIABETES

Nicole: Another aspect of life as a newly independent young adult is shared living space. Many young adults have a stint with a roommate and that means learning to negotiate life, space, stuff, and time with another person—all the time. This can be a stressful experience. Roommates are less forgiving than your family and they often have less history with you.

Adding T1D to the mix can cause tension. This is why extra preparation, consideration and time are necessary for the young adult with T1D when making decisions about living environments.

I have had my share of good and not so good relationship experiences in my life with diabetes. In the less than perfect scenarios, lack of communication and empathy were the root causes of the conflict. In the beginning of any kind of relationship, you should be extra vigilant to assess the other person's capacity to care. You never know when a tricky situation might arise and you may need a little TLC.

Molly has had more than her share of challenging relationship experiences with roommates. Next, she details an instance where her diabetes and her roommates didn't exactly mix.

Roommates
By: Molly Finneran

I have come to believe that the only people in this life that understand the risks associated with my T1D are my parents. You can educate your roommates as much as possible, but they do not love you the way your family does and things can happen that they may not be trained to handle.

I have had diabetes for 21 years, and I am in my final year of pharmacy school in Ohio. For the past two years, I have texted my dad every morning to tell him that I am awake. We do this as a precaution to make sure that I don't have hypoglycemia that prevents me from waking up. I don't enjoy waking up and texting my dad, but it allows me to know that I won't get into trouble and my parents to know that their daughter won't have a coma that she never wakes up from, or worse, dies from.

There is a story to explain why we began this daily text with my dad. It was a weekend and there was a huge snowstorm about to hit the area. I went to sleep on Friday night around 9 pm, and I awoke the next day to my mother calling me—at 3 pm on Saturday afternoon. I had slept nearly 18 hours.

I saw the ambulance outside my apartment. I even told the paramedics that I had juice in my mini-fridge in my room. They checked my blood sugar after I started drinking my juice and it was in the 30s. To this day I'm slightly angry that they gave me the glucagon shot, as I was awake and drinking juice. My blood sugars were in the 500s by 7 pm and I definitely didn't feel that well. Most people in the healthcare profession are trained to know that glucagon should be given when the patient is unconscious or unable to orally take sugar.

During all of this time my roommate was upstairs completely unaware. She never thought that it was strange that I hadn't been awake all day to go to the bathroom or eat breakfast. I was very lucky that my mom had tried to call me. Because of the snowstorm on its way, my school's campus was closed which made her think of me. So that's the story of how I started texting my father every morning: "I'm up. Luv u."

Bullying and Peer Relationships

Nicole: Disclosure about T1D is always a difficult decision. Life should allow for people with challenges to be open about their experience, without judgment. Life isn't always however fair. Sometimes we encounter people who lack sensitivity and tact. Amanda had that experience. I am sure there are many other stories like this one that go untold. It is our combined responsibility to inform, educate, mediate, and, when necessary, litigate to make sure people are respected – no matter the circumstance.

My Challenges with Disclosure in College
By: Amanda Mezer

I have had T1D since I was in 1st grade and I can only recall being teased once shortly after I was diagnosed. Looking back, this boy called me "diabetes girl" and probably wanted attention from the teacher or from me. Then again, that kind of comment is not surprising from a child and I was probably lucky that was the extent of it until I went to college. I have been an advocate for T1D awareness since I was ten, which has made it fairly easy for me to articulate and explain about my disease to others. My expectation has always been that people may ask me questions because I have T1D and I would explain what I could. I had educated hundreds of people over the years: classmates, friends, teachers, and even doctors and nurses. However, when I was in my second year of college, I encountered two roommates/sorority sisters who did not ask questions, but instead went behind my back and spread rumors about me due to their ignorance about T1D. I had told both of my sorority sisters about my T1D the year before when we were selecting roommates. At that time, they voiced no concern and we all happily wanted to room together. After two months of living together, they took their "concerns" about living with me directly to the Dean of Student Affairs, asking that I be removed from the campus housing that I shared with them.

The Dean said these roommates had told him that they could not live under the "circumstances" created by living with someone with diabetes. Yes, that is correct. These girls could not live with me because of my T1D. The accusations included pictures of two test strips on the floor, a picture of my used insulin pump sites in the trash and pictures of blood droppings on the toilet seat, from where they claimed I gave myself shots. As you all know, a test strip is no more harmful than a used Band-Aid, or probably less so since there is such a minute amount of blood residue on each one. We find test strips everywhere from movie theaters to city streets. I had safely disposed of all of the needles that I use in a sharps container that I kept in my closet. I was very careful about making sure the different supplies that were used for my T1D management were disposed of properly. My initial reaction to the photographs was, "where else are the used infusion sites supposed to go other than the trash?"

My roommates asserted that the blood droplets on the toilet were from me giving insulin shots over the toilet. Really?

First, I wear an insulin pump and almost never give any shots. Second, I would never give a shot in a bathroom shared by three people, since it was not that clean and I surely would not be standing over the toilet! Finally, as most everyone knows, insulin shots do not bleed, well, at least not enough to drip. These two roommates clearly knew very little about T1D and chose to remain ignorant and afraid, instead of talking to me about their concerns.

The roommate who shared the same room with me also complained that when my 'insulin pump' beeped during the night, it was disturbing her sleep and she said that she was stressed because she was afraid that the beeping meant that I would die in the middle of the night. The beeping was my CGM sensor alarming me that my blood sugar was either dropping or rising, so I could be warned of a high or a low that would allow me to better manage my blood sugar and prevent a serious problem. I had explained this to her at the beginning of the semester, but she persisted. Sadly, the Dean's office also did not understand this either. The medical director of the Health Center had to confirm this for the Dean at one of the many meetings that occurred as a result of these complaints.

Nicole: In the young adult years relationships tend to be a dominant factor in determining our perspectives. However, remember you have a voice. In this next section we want to discuss healthy relationships and "type 3s." A "type 3" is a person who cares about someone with type 1 or type 2 diabetes. This goes back to the assertion earlier that "Friends are medicine." Finding supportive type 3s is critical – throughout every stage in life.

Romantic Relationships and T1D

Nicole: Type 1 diabetes has an incredible emotional impact not only on me, but also on those who are my "type 3s." There is often huge struggle in the hearts and minds of type 3s. They actually often go through many of the same emotional stages that those with T1D go through. It is important to recognize, however, that no two people go through emotional stages at the same pace.

This is part of the reason why it is so important to talk openly and often about T1D and how we are all coping together. If this is not discussed, it could lead to forms of diabetes and personal sabotage. It can also lead to bitterness and breakup. It doesn't have to be that way.

For example, while you may be feeling relief that you can manage your T1D, your partner or other family members may be afraid or angry at what has happened to you. Or, out of fear, your type 3s may turn into the diabetes police. They don't mean to offend; they are just channeling their concern for the person with T1D in a controlling way. Don't get angry. Use the opportunity to help your type 3s better communicate with you.

Sometimes it is helpful for a physician, counselor, or diabetes educator to talk with the family or loved ones of the person with diabetes. This type of intervention can help with understanding, the development of positive support behaviors, and general understanding or education about diabetes. This can also help alleviate fear and anxiety for the Type 3's.

One of the greatest things I did for my diabetes was ask my loved ones to wear an insulin pump and walk a few days in my shoes. This small action had a big emotional impact and opened the door for great understanding and compassion. When a loved one is willing to physically commit to understanding diabetes, emotional understanding isn't far behind.

Here is what is most important: Everyone in the family needs to feel that they matter and that they are appreciated. This helps with connection to the condition. It also helps diffuse conflict when family members are thanked for their contributions before chided for their wrongdoings.

Teamwork can aid in coping with diabetes and the emotional turmoil that accompanies the condition. Creating an environment of understanding and openness is key. It also helps if there are physical supports. For instance, for many years my parents have a "safe" cabinet in the kitchen that has the healthy "Nicole" foods in it. In our home, the entire family couldn't change habits, but they could make an effort to accommodate the T1D while not forcing complete family change and thus perpetuating family bitterness.

If all parties recognize that with a chronic disease like diabetes there are no simple, quick solutions, life will be much easier. For the person with diabetes, this philosophy will ease anxiety and help make lifestyle adjustments permanent instead of temporary. What I mean is the temptation to go all or nothing is a dead end—it is a losing battle. Slow and steady wins every time.

So maybe you are dating someone or starting to get serious and maybe you are thinking about engaging in an intimate relationship or even taking a bigger step toward commitment, we want to help you have healthy conversations about diabetes with the person who has become your Type 3. The first step is a conversation about needs, wants and barriers with your diabetes.

On **www.studentswithdiabetes.com**, there is a love card that is meant to be a conversation starter to help you and your partner understand the emotions surrounding T1D and the deep meaning of partnership with a person who has T1D. This is a great first step in starting the conversation about diabetes partnership.

It is important to recognize that life with T1D is challenging and because of that it is important to make sure you are with a kind, compassionate, loving, understanding partner who is willing to invest in their own personal understanding of what will be your shared diabetes.

Intimacy and T1D

"If you are not ready to talk to the person you are about to have sex with about sex and diabetes, you are not ready to have sex."

Nicole: Living with diabetes does affect sexual health. This is universal for men and women. The effects are different with age and gender, but the impact is still the same. This section is meant to inform you about how T1D will affect your sexual health and what you might need to consider because of it.

For men, T1D can lead to erectile dysfunction or low testosterone, which can have an impact on your emotional health. Erectile dysfunction (ED) is often related to damage to blood vessels and nerves. This can be related to high blood sugars. There are some lifestyle situations that can also relate to ED. The National Diabetes Information Clearinghouse within the NIH indicates that in addition to diabetes, other health conditions like high blood pressure, kidney disease, alcohol abuse and stress can contribute to ED. (http://diabetes.niddk.nih.gov/dm/pubs/sup/)

The best thing a man with T1D can do is to engage in open dialogue with his partner and his medical team about diabetes and sexual health. Although it can be embarrassing, it is important to talk through symptoms and then investigate potential remedies.

Low testosterone is a common condition that affects over 13 million men. The condition is left untreated in 90 percent of those men. (ADA, ,http://www.diabetes.org/living-with-diabetes/complications/mens-health/sexual-health/low-testosterone.html). The symptoms of low testosterone can include loss of interest in sex, ED, reduced lean body mass, depressed mood, and lack of energy. A simple blood test can tell you if this is a challenge you are facing. The good news is that there are numerous treatment options.

For women, there are also several sexual health side effects of T1D. For many women high blood sugars lead to yeast infections. This uncomfortable situation is common and can be treated easily. The best advice is for women to also have open conversations with their health team about sexual health. Many times, health professionals will work with women who have frequent yeast infections so they have easy access to treatments to make life more bearable.

It is no secret that blood-sugar control changes with hormones. Menstrual cycles often throw diabetes care a whammy. The week before and during menstrual periods are challenging. A word of advice: look for patterns and then set your insulin delivery to match those hormone patterns. Many women on pumps have different pump settings for menstruation because the differences and needs are so significant.

Intimacy and Diabetes
By: Student With Diabetes
"The first time I had sex with my boyfriend I was completely comfortable. We had discussed the implications and understood what it meant for each of us. My boyfriend was very helpful with my diabetes care. At the time, I wore an insulin pump and I decided to disconnect not to be

bothered with the hassle of having a cord and electronic box hanging off my body and tying me to one spot. I personally think this is the way to go if you have a pump... just remember to reconnect! My boyfriend was the one who handed me my pump afterwards and gave me the reminder to put it back on. Admittedly, sometimes if I was going to change a site soon anyway, I'd take it off completely before getting intimate.

Nicole: The story above is representative of a young couple that took the right steps, beginning with open communication. They approached diabetes as a team, talked through the realities of living with T1D, and they decided to be mutually supportive of each other.

Let's get right to it, though—the biggest problem with sex and T1D is that sex is a form of exercise. If you tend to go low when you exercise, you might want to think about how to avoid a similar situation during intimate moments.

Another thing to consider is if your blood sugar is high before intimacy, this could cause ED for guys and vaginal dryness for ladies. Either way, it can be disruptive and potentially difficult and embarrassing.

If you have a sense of humor about it all and have a comfortable, warm, loving relationship with your partner, diabetes doesn't have to get in the way of your relationship. Don't get me wrong, there will be diabetes drama—it happens to everyone. However, when this happens, you will learn quickly if your partner has long-term potential. If they are understanding and helpful, you just might want to think about hanging on to them. If they are accusatory, cold, and annoyed, toss them to the curb. I am blunt because with love comes the opportunity for a baby—and a baby when you have T1D is no walk in the park. This life phase requires a partnership that is strong and well informed, and it requires discipline and a lot of hard work from the mom with diabetes. The end result will be wonderful, but the journey may be a bit tough. Through it all, a good partner is a tremendous asset for the person with T1D.

PREGNANCY WITH T1D

Nicole: My pregnancy experience was amazing. Every aspect of the process was magical, even the delivery. However, the magic can be stolen from a woman with T1D if she doesn't have the proper care, treatment, and management of her T1D before and during her pregnancy.

Let's explore the issue of T1D and pregnancy, and what it takes to ensure both mom and baby are healthy.

When I first started talking about the possibility of having a baby, I was met with all kinds of responses. The range was everywhere from elation to dismay. It seems so many people have the image of the character Shelby from the movie *Steel Magnolias* in their minds when women with T1D talk about pregnancy. (If you don't know, Shelby, a woman with T1D, becomes pregnant, has a child, and shortly thereafter dies from complications of T1D). But the situation need not be so bleak. It is possible to have a wonderfully normal pregnancy, along with a healthy baby, all while managing T1D. But there is a caveat – if a woman with

T1D is not in good control of her blood sugars, tragedy can result. This was the case in *Steel Magnolias*, although subtle in presentation and often not understood by all viewers. Shelby's diabetes care was not optimal and she was having wild glucose swings before her pregnancy.

Create a Team

Success in pregnancy and diabetes starts with the team you have surrounding you. This is not as easy as it may sound. Far before you get pregnant you should interview and organize a team that will help you achieve your goals. Your team should consist of your endocrinologist, registered dietician, diabetes educator and obstetrician or neonatologist. This group will work with you to help you prepare for your pregnancy, and will see you through nine months of incredible diabetes changes. Prior to conception, have a discussion with the physician who will be caring for you. During your meeting, ask questions about how many women with T1D the physician has worked with; the overall health team's experience with insulin and diabetes technology; and the health team's recommended protocols for T1D management during pregnancy, labor, and post-partum. This information will help you determine if the team philosophies are in line with your desires for pregnancy with diabetes.

On a personal note, I changed my health team in the first trimester of my pregnancy because of differences in approach. It is all about finding health professionals that will work with you and I was lucky that in the end I was able to design an ideal team.

During your pregnancy, your doctor visits will consist of several tests including A1cs, urinalysis, thyroid tests, and electrocardiograms for both you and the baby. During my pregnancy, because of the baby and accompanying hormones, my A1c was in the 5 percent range. Don't freak out – this sounds scary, but it is much more doable that you might think. The baby actually helps mom with her blood sugars throughout pregnancy. After delivery, A1c management became much more difficult and tricky, especially during breastfeeding and my A1c levels went back to the 7% range.

Weight Gain

Your healthcare team will direct you regarding your daily behaviors like calorie intake and exercise. Most of the recommendations here are based on a combination of factors including your height, weight, age, and pre-pregnancy activity level. The team will work with you to develop plans so you can maintain an ideal weight and good blood-glucose control. Excessive weight gain is dangerous for women with T1D because the baby gains too much weight, making natural delivery almost impossible. It is recommended that women gain about 20 pounds during pregnancy (National Diabetes Information Clearinghouse - http://www.diabetes.niddk.nih.gov/dm/pubs/pregnancy/#eating).

Exercise

Be sure to talk to your doctor about an exercise program. Exercise is important to all of us, and depending on where you are with your routine when you get pregnant you will receive different advice for exercise throughout pregnancy. Activity is great for the growing baby and it helps the mother maintain good muscle tone and strength throughout pregnancy, which is a benefit during delivery. ☺

My exercise routine varied over the course of my pregnancy. During the first month, I worked out for 60-75 minute sessions 4-5 times a week. But during months two and three, I was so tired I could hardly manage 20 minute walks with my dog. In those same early months, my glucose was so fragile that exercise became an impediment to optimal control and had to be altered to avoid adrenaline highs. In months four and five, I resumed exercise sessions 4-5 times a week and figured out ways to head off highs and lows during and after my workouts. Toward the end of my pregnancy, I was walking about 30 minutes at a time and doing light floor exercises for about 10 minutes every other day. During exercise sessions, I checked my blood sugar 3 times: before exercising, immediately after my cardiovascular workout, and again 15-20 minutes after the entire session ended.

Eye Care

At some points in pregnancy, the mom with T1D can experience some fluctuations in her vision. For this reason, it is recommended that you visit your ophthalmologist for a baseline exam to assess risk for or the presence of retinopathy prior to becoming pregnant. If any laser treatment is necessary, it can be performed prior to getting pregnant. During pregnancy there should be at least two more visits to the ophthalmologist to assess any change in vision or retinopathy symptoms. Diabetic retinopathy can escalate during pregnancy and your vision can change a bit.

During my pregnancy, my eyes did change. My distance vision became worse and I developed the need for glasses. My vision self-corrected after delivery. Scary – yes, doable – yes!

Diabetes Specific Treatment

I will honestly say that my pregnancy would have been a nightmare without the insulin pump. I realize there are plenty of women who do well with injection therapy, however I don't think I would be one of them. My insulin dosage changed weekly and the pump allowed me the flexibility I needed to micromanage my diabetes care and still enjoy the foods I was used to and craving. Today, sensors are an incredible asset for T1D women who are planning to be or already are pregnant. The goal is to keep blood sugars very tightly managed and the sensor and pump help women do just that. The morale of this story is to use all the tools available to you.

Research

I was fortunate to work with one of the world leaders in T1D and pregnancy, Dr. Lois Jovanovic, (Sansum Diabetes Institute, Santa Barbara, CA) when I was carrying my little one. During our partnership, she invited me to participate in fascinating research that could hold potential keys to the mystery of diabetes in general. Amazingly, about 25 percent of pregnant women with T1D create and use a portion of their own insulin during the pregnancy period. It is speculated that these women thrive off of the mild immunosuppressive state and the growth hormones being produced by the placenta.

Specifically, these women show a rise in their C-peptide levels and a drop in their insulin requirements. So far, the C-peptide rise has been parallel to a rise in pregnancy-related growth factors (prolactin and placental lactogen), and the pregnancy-related immunosuppressive hormones (cortisol and progesterone).

This research empowered me and taught me to participate in T1D research in ways I had not before. Sadly, the insulin creation during pregnancy ended for me shortly after delivery, but what an incredible experience to be a part of such interesting medical research. You can find out more about opportunities for you to participate in research by investigating trials.jdrf.org. I encourage you to think about how you might be able to be a part of the solution to diabetes by participating in diabetes research in your area.

Genetics

One of the emotionally traumatic aspects of pregnancy is the concern about genetics and the risk for the baby. The Joslin Diabetes Center offers comprehensive information on diabetes risk and is a good resource for gathering more information than what is offered in the next few paragraphs. You can find information at: http://www.joslin.org/info/genetics_and_diabetes.html.

In general, if an immediate relative has T1D, one's risk of developing T1D is 10 to 20 times the risk of the general population. A lot depends on which parent has T1D. The risk for the child developing T1D is lower if the mother has T1D, as opposed to the father. If you are a woman with T1D and your child was born before you were 25, your child's risk is 1 in 25; if your child was born after you turned 25, your child's risk is 1 in 100, the same for most Americans. Don't let statistics scare you though. If you have questions or concerns, talk to your health team about the risks and options. (http://www.joslin.org/info/genetics_and_diabetes.html)

Breastfeeding

Nicole: One of the most difficult parts of having my baby came after she was born. Yes, the pain of labor and delivery was intense, but the frustration and the not knowing associated with caring for the baby, specifically breastfeeding, was even more painful. There are so many complications or challenges associated with breast-feeding for women with T1D and their babies. In the first few days, my frustration was mainly in learning what to do. And that frustration applied to both the baby and me.

Although difficult, I was committed to breastfeeding for the recommended six months (Stuebe, 2007). My motivation came from research. I wanted to do all I could to make sure this baby had the best start in life but I also wanted to make sure that I did all I could to help the baby avoid a diagnosis of T1D. Some scientists have speculated that there is a correlation between T1D, breastfeeding, and cow's milk product introduction. That speculation is the reason my baby and I entered the research study TRIGR (Trial to Reduce IDDM in the Genetically at Risk). The aim was to help find out what that correlation is and how to prevent T1D.

There was some risk in my decision to be involved. Participation meant the baby and I would be randomized in the trial for the formula supplementation. The caveat is that it is up to the mother if the formula will be used or not. Mothers could choose to breastfeed exclusively if they desired. I knew, however, that I would not have that luxury. With plans to resume work and travel when the baby reached two months, supplementation was most definitely in my future.

Our study results were encouraging, as my little one did not have the genetic risk to continue in the trial. Infants needed to be in a higher risk category for continued research. Our elimination, only encouraged me to participate as if I was a study member.

The Trial to Reduce Insulin Dependent Diabetes in the Genetically at Risk (TRIGR) is an international study with the goal of determining whether using special formula or breast milk, rather than cow's milk, during the first 6-8 months of life can prevent or delay T1D in children who have an increased genetic risk.

Breastfeeding has many other complicating elements outside of formula choice. I didn't expect or plan on the psychological turmoil I experienced associated with breastfeeding and T1D.

During the first month, at one point when I fed the baby, I didn't know my blood sugar was extremely high. It was over 300 after I had finished the feeding. I was panicked and terrified. All I could do was cry. Had I hurt the baby? I called my doctor immediately and received advice on what to do. She instructed me to pump out all the milk in my breasts and discard it. She told me the baby would be fussy for the next few hours because her pancreas would be working extra hard to deal with the extra sugar in her system and the baby would be at risk for thrush (yeast infection in her mouth). It was so upsetting, and yes, the baby did cry for hours and had a mild case of thrush!

I didn't even think about this scenario before the baby. All I had heard about were low blood sugars during feedings. Typically during feedings, the baby is taking so much from the mother's system that the mother's glucose drops. I was on edge about that scenario and the danger it could pose to the baby, not the reverse. Now, I had plenty of lows during feedings and it turns out those are easy to deal with. I usually fed the baby in a large chair next to a supply of juice boxes, Gatorade, and peanut butter crackers. Before each feeding I learned to test my blood sugar to make sure I was okay and was starting the feed in a good glucose range. If my blood sugar was low or nearing the low range, I would treat it with something from my supply. Typically, during each session I would drink one box of juice or one Gatorade.

Sometimes the challenge and the guilt associated with blood sugar numbers and feeding the baby made me want to stop breastfeeding. It often seemed too difficult, too time consuming, and too dangerous for my child. However, I did continue for seven months, with enough milk frozen to continue feeding the baby with breast milk through the eighth month. I finally stopped because of my dwindling milk production and work schedule. I am proud that I was able to provide for my child and hopefully provide her immunity that will protect her in the long run.

FINDING BALANCE

Nicole: If often seems as though life should get a speeding ticket, because it is racing forward so fast that we can hardly catch our breath. As a person with T1D, I struggle with the tendency to live from meal to meal and glucose check to glucose check. Sometimes, the intensity of disease management can steal the enjoyment out of life. "Can" is the most important word there—it can steal joy, but it doesn't have to. Each of us is the author of our own life script. We determine our potential. We can find balance between life, family, career, community, and T1D. That doesn't mean it is or will be easy, but it is possible.

In my harried life, I have found five keys that help me manage and enjoy the most of every moment. I hope these tips will help you find peace and balance in your life with T1D.

The first key to success is the presence of **relationships**. Loving support offers confidence for the person with diabetes. When one feels confident, one feels supported and therefore has a measure of balance in life. The lack of relationships leaves one in isolation, with little support, and the likelihood of self-doubt, self- loathing, and depression.

Loving support alone isn't the answer. **Categorical thinking** is my next key to finding balance. I have found that as a mother, professional, student, and a person with T1D I have to section off my day to accomplish all that I desire and that others need from me. It helps me to write lists and to categorize my responsibilities. Make time for your T1Ds or else T1D will take time away from you.

That is the third key is **flexibility** or the ability to give you permission to not be perfect. Don't pressure yourself to get it all right all the time. There has to be a measure of flexibility in your approach. If you don't exercise every day, that is okay. Making the effort to be more active than not is the key. Forward momentum deserves reward. The same is true for food and glucose checking. No one is going to get everything perfect all the time. This is one of the most difficult traits to master, particularly in a society that praises perfection. If you have a perfection expectation, you are setting yourself up for disappointment. We don't want that to happen.

The fourth key is to have an **attitude of acceptance**. Allow others to help you. Allowing friends or family to care about you, or even for you, is an important trait to master. This not only helps life operate more smoothly, but it also strengthens relationships.

Finally, the fifth key to balance is the **overarching attitude you bring to life**. Are you living a life of optimism or pessimism? The way you see the world and your place in it has a tremendous impact on your T1D. Identifying your reason for living and therefore the reason to care for your T1D is crucial. It is difficult to live with T1D and to balance diabetes care with the other responsibilities of life. In the difficulty, though, there is incredible joy, should you choose to see it.

Giving Back

Nicole: My attitude toward life and diabetes is one of enduring gratefulness. This approach allows me the freedom to expel any negative feelings with the knowledge that every day is a gift, even with diabetes. I am blessed to survive a disease that 100 years ago was unbeatable. It is by the grace of God that I work in an arena that is focused on serving others. This attitude is the secret to my success. Students With Diabetes, the young adult organization I founded, is meant to serve a population that is often forgotten. It is meant to provide a safe place for young adults as they explore adulthood and decide about their future. It is meant to teach young adults about the power of relationships. I bring this up to serve as an example. Living with T1D brings great experience and value if you choose to see it that way. It is a choice. Opportunity abounds for those who are willing to see diabetes through the lens of hope and service.

For those who love a T1D: by being a knowledgeable, non-judgmental and supportive Type 3, you can make living with diabetes that much easier for the person you care about, ultimately leading to a long, happy, and most of all successful life with diabetes for the entire family.

*If you would like to learn more about Students With Diabetes, visit www.studentswithdiabetes.com. You can start a chapter of this organization in your town or at your school. You can also be a part of the SWD National Internship Program and participate in the National Students With Diabetes Conferences.

ABOUT THE AUTHOR
www.nicolejohnson.com

Nicole Johnson, DrPH, MPH, MA has been living with T1D since 1993 and spends much of her time working on the behalf of people who live with her shared chronic disease. Since her year as Miss America 1999, she has raised over $26 million for diabetes research and programs.

She serves the diabetes community in any way she can from public speaking, to writing, to serving on boards and councils. Presently, Nicole serves on the Florida Governor's Diabetes Advisory Council, the JDRF International Board of Directors and the Tampa Bay JDRF Board of Directors. She is a past national board member for the American Diabetes Association and a past appointee to the National Institutes of Health Council of Public Representatives.

Nicole is a Telly award-winning television journalist and an avid writer. Her articles on living with T1D have appeared in *Guideposts* magazine, *Diabetes Forecast*, *Diabetes Health*, *USA Today*, and on various websites related to diabetes. She has written six books, including her autobiography *Living with Diabetes* and her most recent cookbook *Nicole Johnson's Diabetes Recipe Makeovers*.

Nicole serves as the Executive Director of Bringing Science Home, at the University of South Florida, a research program focused on helping people with diabetes live better lives. Within this program Nicole founded a national organization called Students With Diabetes that serves young adults with Type 1 Diabetes and their Type 3's.

Nicole holds master's degrees in journalism and public health, as well as a doctorate in public health.

WORKS CITED

American Diabetes Association. "The Health Insurance Marketplace & People with Diabetes: American Diabetes Association®." Retrieved from http://www.diabetes.org/living-with-diabetes/health-insurance/health-insurance-marketplace.html

American Diabetes Association. "Low Testosterone in Men With Diabetes." Retrieved from http://www.diabetes.org/living-with-diabetes/treatment-and-care/men/low-testosterone.html

American With Disabilities Amendments Act of 2008 (ADA).

Americans With Disabilities Amendment Act of 2008, Statement of the Manager's to Accompany S. 3406.

Bandura, A. (1997). Self-efficacy: The exercise of control. New York: Freeman.

Bevans, K. B., Riley, A. W., Moon, J., & Forrest, C. B. (2010). Conceptual and methodological advances in child-reported outcomes measurement. Expert Review of Pharmacoeconomics & Outcomes Research, 10(40), 385-96.

Compton, William C. (2005). An Introduction to Positive Psychology. Wadsworth Publishing. pp. 1–22. ISBN 0-534-64453-8.

EEOC Home Page. "EEOC Home Page." Retrieved from www.eeoc.gov

Edede L.E. & Ellis C. (2010). Diabetes and depression: global perspectives. Diabetes Res Clin Pract.; 87(3):302-12.

Emmons & McCullough, (2003). Counting blessings versus burdens: an experimental investigation of gratitude and subjective well-being in daily life. J Pers Soc Psychol; 84(2):377-89.

Johnson, Nicole. (2010). Nicole Johnson's Diabetes Recipe Makeovers. Lincolnwood, IL: Publications International.

Joslin Diabetes Center. "Genetics & Diabetes: What's Your Risk?" Genetics & Diabetes: What's Your Risk? Retrieved from www.joslin.org/info/genetics_and_diabetes.html

Kyngas, H. Hentinen, M. Barlow, J. (1998). Adolescents Perceptions of Physicians, Nurses, Parents and Friends: Help or Hindrance in Compliance with Diabetes Self-Care? Journal of Advanced Nursing; 27: 760-769.

Li, Ford, Strine, & Mokdad, (2008). Diabetes and anxiety in US adults: findings from the 2006 Behavioral Risk Factor Surveillance System. Diabetic Medicine.

Lyubomirsky, Sonja (2007). The How of Happiness. London: Sphere.

Lyubomirsky, Tkach, & Sheldon (2004). The Case for Altruism. Authentic Happiness, University of Pennsylvania Newsletter.

Lykken, David T. and Tellegen, Auke (1996). Happiness is a Stochastic Phenomenon.

McCormick."Edamame and Corn Salad with Oregano Vinaigrette Recipe." Retrieved from www.mccormick.com

National Diabetes Information Clearinghouse (NDIC). "Sexual and Urologic Problems of Diabetes." Retrieved from http://diabetes.niddk.nih.gov/dm/pubs/sup/

National Diabetes Information Clearinghouse (NDIC). "What I Need to Know about Preparing for Pregnancy If I Have Diabetes." Retrieved from http://www.diabetes.niddk.nih.gov/dm/pubs/pregnancy/

Osborn, C.Y. & Egede L.E. Validation of an Information-Motivation-Behavioral Skills model of diabetes self-care (IMB-DSC). Patient education and counseling. 2010; 79: 49-54.

Rasmussen H.N., Scheier M.F., Greenhouse JB. (2009). Optimism and physical health: a meta-analytic review. Ann Behav Med; 37(3):239-56.

Sheldon, B.H. & Quin, MB. (2005). Practical Diabetes International; 22(6), 222-224.

Sheldon, K.M., Kasser, T., Smith, K., & Share, T. (2002). Personal goals and psychological growth: Testing an intervention to enhance goal-attainment and personality integration. Journal of Personality, 70, 5-31.

Stuebe. A. (2007), Breastfeeding and diabetes – benefits and special needs. Diabetes Voice. 52:26–9. 13.

Veenhoven, R. (2008). Healthy Happiness: effects of happiness on physical health and the consequences for preventive health care. Journal of Happiness Studies; 9(3). 449-469.

APPENDIX

Below are some of the resources that are helpful to find information about diabetes education, advocacy and programs.

A. **Useful Web Resources:**

- American Diabetes Association: www.diabetes.org
- Behavioral Diabetes Institute: www.behavioraldiabetesinstitute.org
- Bringing Science Home: www.bringingsciencehome.com
- Centers for Disease Control and Prevention (CDC): www.cdc.gov
- Children With Diabetes: www.childrenwithdiabetes.com
- Clinical Trials Connection: http://trials.jdrf.org
- Diabetes Daily: www.diabetesdaily.com
- Diabetes Hands Foundation: www.diabeteshandsfoundation.org
- Diabetes Health: www.diabeteshealth.com
- Diabetes Mine: www.diabetesmine.com
- Diabetes Scholars Foundation: www.diabetesscholars.org
- Diabetes Self-Management: www.diabetesselfmanagement.com
- Diabetes Sisters: www.diabetessisters.org
- Diabetically Speaking: www.diabeticallyspeaking.com
- dLife: www.dlife.com
- International Diabetes Federation: www.idf.org
- IDF Young Leaders Program: www.idf.org/young-leaders-programme
- JDRF: www.jdrf.org
- National Institutes of Health (NIH): www.nih.gov
- National Institute of Diabetes and Digestive and Kidney Diseases (NIDDK): www.niddk.nih.gov
- Online Diabetes Support Team: http://jdrf.org/life-with-t1d/get-support/
- PADRE Foundation: www.padrefoundation.org
- Scott's Diabetes: www.scottsdiabetes.com
- Six Until Me: www.sixuntilme.com
- Students With Diabetes: www.studentswithdiabetes.com
- TuDiabetes: www.tudiabetes.org

B. **Places to Get Diabetes Supplies without Insurance:**

- Financial Help for Diabetes Care (NIH): http://diabetes.niddk.nih.gov/dm/pubs/financialhelp/index.aspx
- Partnership for Prescription Assistance: www.pparx.org
- RxAssist: rxassist.org
- Together RX Access Card: www.togetherrxaccess.com

C. Health Insurance Information:

- cms.gov/MedicaidEligibility/
- healthcare.gov/
- healthinsurancefinders.com/cr_state_department_of_insurance.ht ml
- medicaid.gov/ health-insurance.org/getting-started
- nlm.nih.gov/medlineplus/healthinsurance.html
  http://www.ahrq.gov/questions/

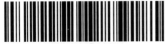

Made in the USA
San Bernardino, CA
09 January 2018